KOY KUT

# 6 Steps to Healthy Hair

*Hair Care Tips to grow your natural hair long and healthy.*

*To everyone who's ever stood in front of the mirror wondering*
*what went wrong —*
*this is for you.*
*To the ones who've tried every product, every style, every shortcut,*
*and still felt like their hair just wouldn't cooperate —*
*this book is your fresh start.*
*To every young person learning to love what naturally grows from*
*their head,*
*and to every adult finally unlearning everything they were taught*
*about "good hair,"*
*this is for the journey back to understanding yourself.*

"When you understand your hair, you understand your roots — and when you understand your roots, you grow differently."

— Koy Kut

# Contents

# Foreword

When it comes to hair, most people only see what's on the surface — a style, a color, a vibe. But hair is more than that. It's how we express ourselves, how we show up to the world, and for many of us, how we feel about who we are. I've seen it firsthand — the confidence boost after a clean cut, the way someone's energy shifts after a fresh twist, or the quiet power that comes from finally understanding your own hair.

That's what this book is about — understanding.

Because hair care isn't just about products, it's about *knowledge*. It's about knowing how your scalp works, how your strands behave, and how to build a relationship with your hair instead of fighting against it. Once you understand the "why" behind what your hair does, you stop chasing trends and start creating routines that actually work for you.

I wrote **"6 Steps to Healthy Hair"** not as a rulebook, but as a guide — one that simplifies the science and replaces confusion with clarity. Whether you're rocking locs, coils, waves, or curls, these steps will help you learn what your hair needs, when it needs it, and how to give it that care without overcomplicating things.

The truth is, healthy hair doesn't happen overnight — it happens when you start paying attention.

Every wash, every detangle, every oiling moment adds up. It's the consistency that brings transformation.

So as you go through these pages, take your time. Experiment. Learn. Unlearn.

Because your hair isn't something to "fix" — it's something to understand, nurture, and celebrate.

Let's get to the root of it — literally.

**— Koy Kut**

# Preface

I didn't write this book to sell another "miracle routine."

I wrote it because I got tired of watching people lose confidence in their natural hair — not because it was unhealthy, but because they didn't understand it.

As a barber and hair specialist, I've seen it all — from heat damage to over-conditioning, from product overload to neglect. But underneath it all, what I've really seen is confusion. People using ten different products without knowing what their hair actually needs. People chasing results that don't match their texture, porosity, or lifestyle.

That's when I realized something simple but powerful: **most hair problems don't start with the hair — they start with a lack of knowledge.**

So I built this book around the basics.

Six steps that anyone can follow — not because they're trendy, but because they work.

Steps that break down how your scalp functions, how your strands react, and how to build a consistent system that finally makes sense.

This book is for the person tired of starting over every few months.

It's for the one who wants healthy hair but doesn't have time for twenty-step routines.

It's for the parent trying to learn their child's hair, the stylist trying to educate clients, or anyone standing in front of a mirror asking, "What's missing?"

You'll find science here — but it won't sound like a textbook.

You'll find technique — but it won't feel complicated.

And you'll find truth — the kind that cuts through marketing and myths to help you rebuild your relationship with your hair.

This is more than just a guide — it's a conversation between you and your roots.

Because once you understand your hair, everything else falls into place.

— **Koy Kut**

# 1

# Scalp and Hair

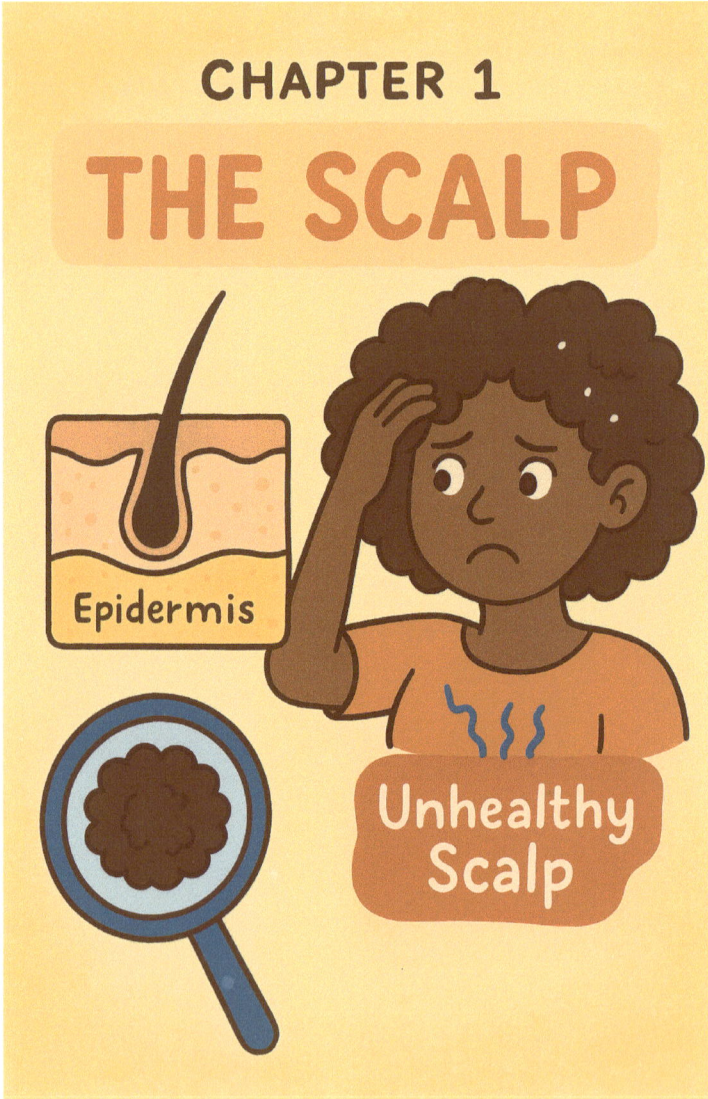

# CHAPTER 1
# THE SCALP

Epidermis

Unhealthy Scalp

Before you can talk about healthy hair, you have to understand where it comes from. Think of your head as a garden. The scalp is the soil. Your hair strands are the plants. Just like in a garden, if the soil is weak, dry, or packed down, the plants struggle. If the soil is rich and watered, the plants thrive.

## The Scalp — The Soil Beneath the Garden

Your scalp is living skin, not just a base for hair. It has two layers:

- **Epidermis (top layer):** The surface you can see and touch. If you notice flakes, redness, or itching, that's your soil telling you it's off balance.
- **Dermis (deep layer):** This is where the roots (hair follicles) sit. Tiny blood vessels feed them, delivering the nutrients your hair needs to grow.

**Signs of an unhealthy scalp:**

- Constant flakes or dandruff
- Itchiness or soreness
- A greasy yet irritated feeling
- Strange smell or buildup that won't go away

**Quick Tip:** Treat your scalp like skin. Don't scrub it raw or cake it with product. Keep it clean, hydrated, and massaged so blood can flow freely.

## Blood Flow — The Water Supply

Plants need steady water to survive. Your follicles need steady blood flow. That blood brings oxygen and nutrients to keep hair in its growth cycle. Poor circulation is like cutting off the water hose — growth slows.

   **Trick:** A one-minute scalp massage in the shower can help stimulate growth. Exercise, good sleep, and drinking water also boost blood flow.

## Hair Strands — The Plants in the Garden

Every strand of hair growing from your scalp is like a little plant. How each strand behaves depends on its traits:

- **Color:** Determined by natural pigment, like flower colors.
- **Density:** The number of strands on your head. Some have a forest, others a smaller patch.
- **Elasticity:** How far hair can stretch without snapping. Healthy hair bounces back, damaged hair breaks.
- **Porosity:** How well your hair absorbs and keeps moisture. High porosity hair is like a sponge (soaks up water fast, loses it fast). Low porosity is like a waxy leaf (hard to get water in).

**Story:** A client once told me, "I moisturize every day, but my hair still feels dry." She had high porosity hair — like a sponge with holes. Once we added a sealing oil after her moisturizer, the water stopped slipping away and her hair finally stayed soft.

4

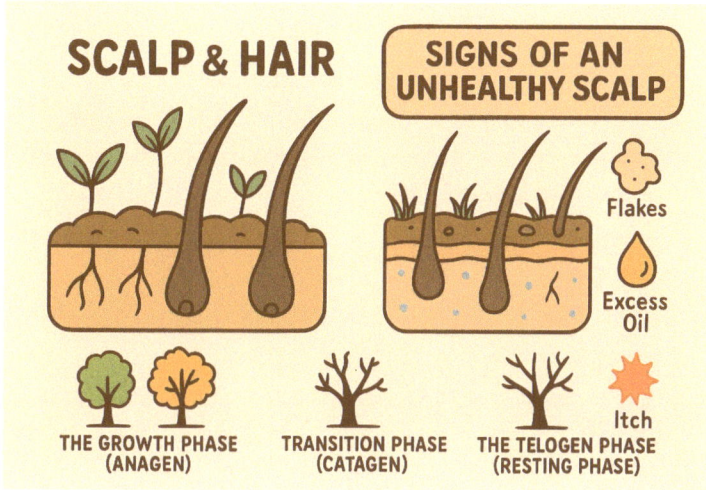

## Growth Cycle — Seasons of Hair

Your hair works in seasons, not nonstop.

- **Anagen (growth):** The active season, like spring and summer. Most of your strands are here.
- **Catagen (transition):** Growth slows down, like fall.
- **Telogen (resting and shedding):** Old hairs fall to make room for new ones, like winter leaves dropping.

**Tip:** Losing hair daily is normal. It's like leaves falling off trees — a sign of life, not death. If you're losing clumps or seeing bald spots, that's when it's time to look closer.

## Takeaways

- A healthy scalp is the base for healthy hair.
- Blood flow feeds follicles, just like water feeds plants.
- Hair strands have unique traits (density, elasticity, porosity) that affect how they behave.
- Growth happens in cycles. Shedding is part of the process.

# 2

# The Secret 6 Steps

Healthy hair isn't about chasing the newest product. It's about sticking to a simple routine that works, the same way a garden thrives with water, sunlight, and protection. Here are the six steps that keep your hair thriving.

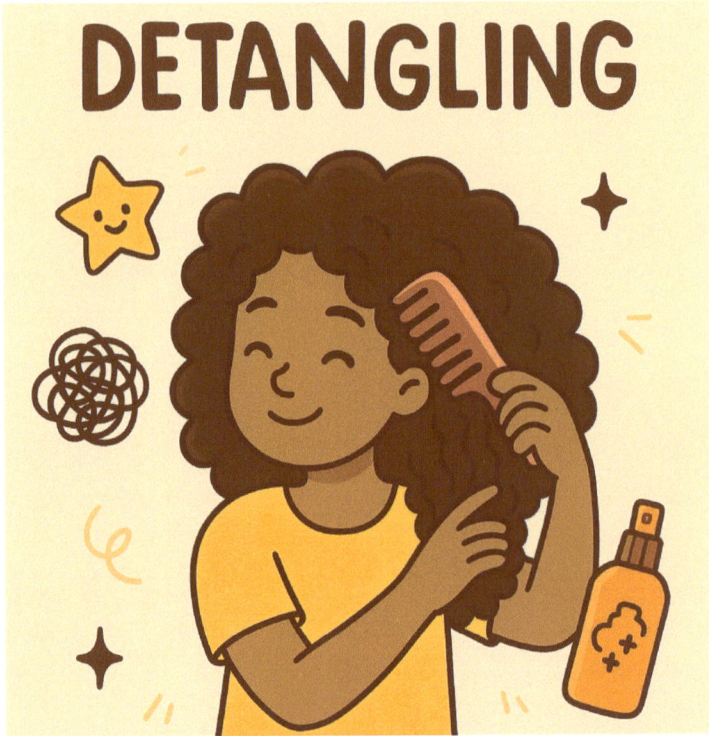

## Step 1: Detangle — Clearing the Path

Think of detangling like clearing weeds out of a garden path. If you yank too hard, you tear up the plants. Hair is the same way — rough detangling leads to breakage.

- **How to do it right:**
- Mist your hair with water or a leave-in before touching it.
- Start at the ends and work upward.
- Use your fingers or a wide-tooth comb.

**Story:** A client once told me she hated wash day because detangling took forever. She used to rip through dry tangles with a fine comb. Once I showed her how to section her hair, spray it down, and finger-detangle first, she cut her detangling time in half — and her breakage almost disappeared.

**Quick Trick:** Hold each section firmly near the root while detangling. That way, you don't tug on the scalp.

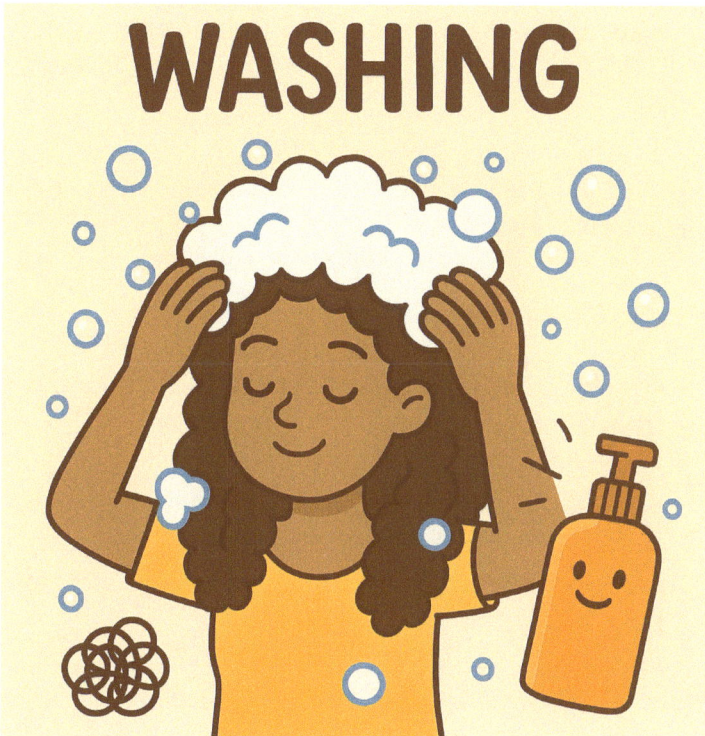

## Step 2: Wash — Refreshing the Soil

Your scalp builds up dirt, oil, sweat, and product — just like soil gathers weeds and debris. Washing clears the ground so hair can grow better.

- **Frequency:** For many, once a week is plenty. If you work out a lot, you may need a midweek rinse or co-wash.
- **Focus:** Massage the scalp with the pads of your fingers. Don't scrub the hair length; let the suds run down.
- **Water temp:** Warm water cleanses, cool water seals the cuticle. Avoid scalding hot showers — they dry everything out.

**Tip:** Pre-poo with oil or conditioner before shampooing to protect fragile ends.

## Step 3: Condition — Feeding the Roots

After washing, your hair is like soil after rain — clean, but thirsty. Conditioner is the fertilizer that restores balance.

- **Rinse-out conditioner:** Adds slip and softness in minutes.
- **Deep conditioner:** Weekly or biweekly, it's a full recharge. Add heat or steam for extra absorption if you have low-porosity hair.

**Story:** I had a client whose curls always looked limp. She thought she needed more gel. Truth was, her hair was over-moisturized and lacked protein. Once we balanced her deep treatments with a monthly protein mask, her curls had bounce again.

**Pro Tip:** Alternate between moisture-based and protein-based conditioners for balance.

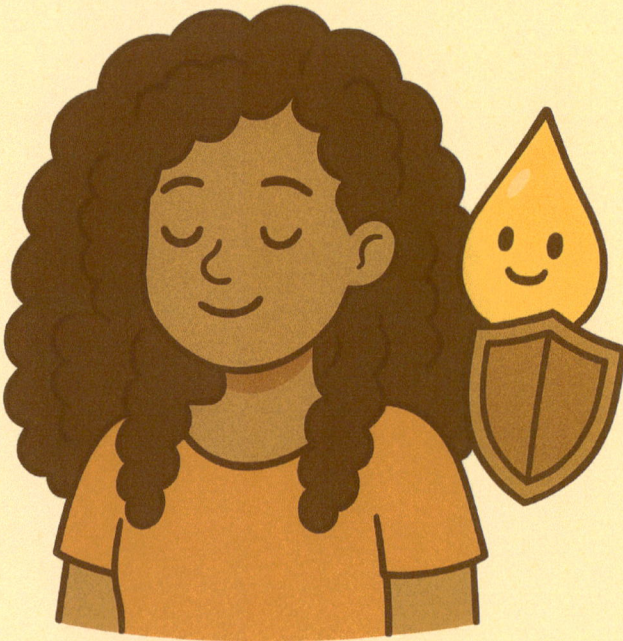

# SEALING

## Step 4: Seal — Locking the Gate

Moisture doesn't last forever unless you seal it in. Oils and butters work like a lid on a water bucket.

- **For fine hair:** Use light oils like grapeseed or jojoba.
- **For thick or porous hair:** Use heavier oils like castor or shea butter blends.

**Tip:** If your hair feels greasy and heavy, you used too much. Sealing should lock in hydration, not drown your hair.

## Step 5: Protect — Building the Fence

You wouldn't leave your garden open to stray animals. Same with your hair — protection keeps it safe.

- **At night:** Use satin or silk pillowcases, bonnets, or scarves. Cotton robs moisture.
- **During the day:** Avoid styles that pull too tight on edges.
- **With heat:** Always use a protectant and stick to moderate temps.

**Truth:** Styles that hurt aren't protective. If it's painful, it's harmful.

## Step 6: Moisturize — Daily Watering

Plants don't survive from one thunderstorm; they need regular watering. Same with your hair — keep it hydrated between wash days.

- **Refresh:** Use a spray bottle with water and a little leave-in.
- **Don't soak:** A mist is enough. Constant drenching weakens hair.
- **Listen:** If hair feels rough, it needs moisture. If it feels soft but limp, it might need protein.

**Story:** A client once drenched her hair every morning thinking more water = more health. Her strands kept breaking. Once she switched to misting lightly, her hair stayed hydrated and strong.

## Takeaways

- Detangle gently from ends to roots.
- Wash often enough to clear buildup but not strip moisture.
- Condition to restore strength and softness.
- Seal to lock in hydration.
- Protect with smart styling and nighttime care.
- Moisturize consistently, not excessively.

# 3

# What Damages Hair

Healthy hair can still fall apart if you don't protect it. Think of a garden: you can water and feed your plants, but if pests, storms, or careless footsteps keep hitting them, they'll never thrive. Hair is the same — damage often comes from what we do without even noticing.

# Risks & Damage

## ✓ Do

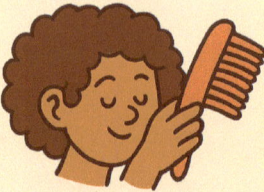

**Gently detangle**

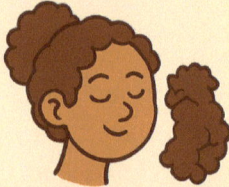

**Wear loose styles**

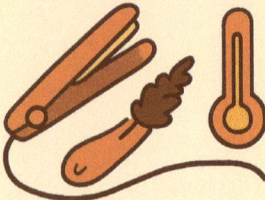

**Use low heat**

## ✕ Don't

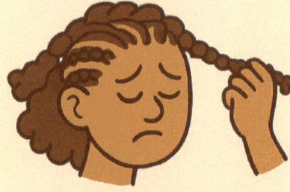

**Roughly comb**

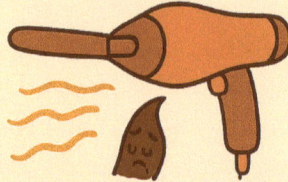

**Apply high heat**

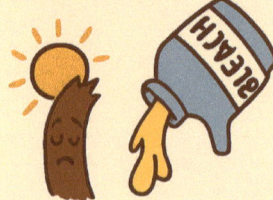

**Use harsh chemicals**

## Chemical Damage — Too Much Too Fast

Bleach, relaxers, dyes, and perms are like pouring acid on your garden fence. They lift the roof tiles (cuticles) on your hair and strip away natural strength.

- **Signs:** Hair feels rough, breaks easily, color fades fast.
- **Tip:** Space out chemical services. Give your hair recovery time with protein and deep moisture.
- **Story:** I had a client who bleached her curls three times in two months. The color was popping, but her hair started snapping like dry twigs. We cut back, added protein treatments, and gave her hair months of recovery before touching color again.

## Physical Damage — Rough Handling

Yanking a brush through tangles, using cheap elastics, or keeping tight braids for weeks is like stepping on young plants over and over. Eventually, they snap.

- **Signs:** Tender scalp, thinning edges, broken pieces around the sink or floor.
- **Tips:**
- Use wide-tooth combs or fingers.
- Switch to scrunchies or covered bands.
- Rotate styles to give edges a break.

**Trick:** If a style hurts when it's fresh, it's too tight. Pain is your hair's way of saying stop.

## Heat Damage — Frying the Garden

Flat irons, blow dryers, and curling wands are like constant sunburn on your plants. One session doesn't destroy everything, but over time, heat weakens your strands.

- **Signs:** Hair won't curl back, feels stiff or stringy after straightening.
- **Tips:**
- Always use a heat protectant.
- Keep temps moderate (300–350°F for most).
- One pass with the iron is better than five.

**Story:** A client came in asking why her curls weren't coming back after months of weekly straightening. We had to cut the heat-damaged ends. Now, she only straightens on special occasions — and her curls bounce again.

## Environmental Damage — Weather and Lifestyle

Wind, sun, chlorine, and even dry indoor air can beat up your hair like storms hitting crops.

- **Signs:** Dryness, tangles, faded color, brittle ends.
- **Tips:**
- Cover hair in harsh weather.
- Rinse and deep condition after swimming.
- Use a humidifier in winter to fight dry air.

## Common Hair Problems — Warning Flags

- **Dandruff vs. Dry Scalp:** Big, oily flakes = dandruff (scalp imbalance). Tiny white flakes = dryness.
- **Chronically Dry Hair:** Often from harsh shampoos or skipping conditioner.
- **Split Ends & Breakage:** Splits travel up the strand if not trimmed.
- **Excessive Shedding:** More than usual over weeks could signal stress, diet, or health issues.
- **Traction Alopecia:** Thinning edges from tight braids, ponytails, or loc retwists.
- **Knots & Tangles:** Common with curly/coily textures. Prevent by moisturizing and keeping ends stretched or tucked at night.

**Pro Tip:** Don't wait until the problem is big. Small trims, gentle handling, and a consistent routine stop most issues before they get serious.

## Takeaways

- Chemicals, heat, and tension are the main enemies of healthy hair.
- Bad habits cause more damage than bad products.
- Pain is a warning sign — listen to your scalp.
- Most damage can be prevented with gentle care and consistency.

# 4

# Chemical Damage

## When Hair Needs Rehab

Chemical damage is like when you push something past its limit.
Think about a favorite pair of jeans: wear them too much, wash
them too rough, bleach them, and eventually the fabric thins,
tears, or loses its stretch. Hair is the same way. Every bleach,
relaxer, dye, or perm works by cracking open the fabric of your
strands and forcing it to change. It's powerful, but it's never
free.

# CHEMICAL DAMAGE

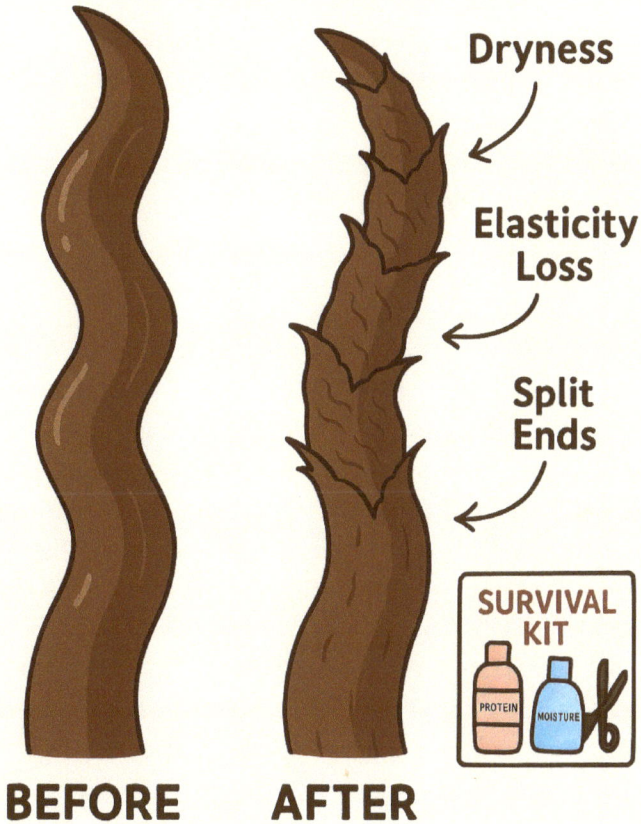

Dryness

Elasticity Loss

Split Ends

SURVIVAL KIT

PROTEIN    MOISTURE

**BEFORE**    **AFTER**

## What Damage Looks Like

Your hair strand is like a rope made of tiny twisted fibers. Chemicals untwist those fibers to change the shape or color. Once the twist is gone, the rope never feels the same again. That's why chemically stressed hair feels:

- **Rough like sandpaper** instead of smooth.
- **Stretchy like chewing gum** when wet, then snapping when you pull.
- **Dull like washed-out fabric** instead of shiny.
- **Sticky and tangled like Velcro**, because the cuticle isn't flat anymore.

That's your strand waving a red flag.

## Why It Happens

Think of your hair like a sponge wrapped in plastic wrap (the cuticle). Bleach, relaxers, and dyes poke holes in that wrap to get inside the sponge. The more holes you make, the weaker the wrap becomes — water leaks out, and the sponge starts to crumble.

The tricky part? You can't just "rewrap" it. Once those holes are there, they stay. That's why repair isn't about *erasing* the damage, it's about patching, protecting, and making the sponge last as long as possible.

## Managing the Damage

Here's where people go wrong: they either overload their hair with protein until it's stiff as straw, or drown it in moisture until it's limp. Damaged hair needs both — like fabric that's torn and also dried out.

- **Protein is the patch kit.** Hydrolyzed keratin, silk, wheat protein — these slip into the cracks and give the strand some strength back.
- **Moisture is the flexibility.** Aloe, honey, glycerin, and deep conditioners keep the strand bendy so it doesn't snap.

Together, protein and moisture act like a tailor sewing up a ripped shirt and then softening the fabric so it drapes right again.

## Protect Like It's Fragile

Imagine your hair is fine silk. You wouldn't throw silk in a hot dryer or scrub it with harsh soap, right? Same with damaged hair:

- **Heat:** Keep it low and rare. Flat irons on damaged hair are like ironing a hole in your favorite shirt — it only gets worse.
- **Combing:** Wide-tooth combs, finger detangling, and slip. No yanking.
- **Night Care:** Satin pillowcase or bonnet. Cotton is like sandpaper on weak strands.
- **Ends:** Seal them with oils or butters, like waxing old wood so it doesn't splinter.

## What You Can't Skip

Split ends don't heal. They're like a run in stockings — once it starts, it only climbs higher. Trimming is your reset button. It doesn't mean giving up on length — it means protecting the length you still have.

And yes, bond builders like Olaplex or K18 can help reconnect some broken links inside the hair. Think of them like glue on a cracked mug: the mug still has a crack, but it holds together longer.

## Story From the Chair

A client once came in after bleaching her hair at home. When I touched it, it felt soft and mushy when wet, then brittle when dry. I explained:

**"Your sponge has too many holes. We can't make it brand new again, but we can make it hold water better and stop it from crumbling."**

We cut off the worst ends, gave her a protein mask for strength, followed with a moisturizing deep conditioner, and sealed it in. Two months later she said, "It's not perfect, but my hair actually feels alive again."

## The Big Lesson

Chemical damage doesn't mean your hair is ruined forever. It means it needs rehab — balance, protection, and patience. Treat it like fabric: patch it, soften it, and protect it until the fresh, undamaged material grows in.

Because the truth is, healthy hair isn't about never taking risks. It's about knowing how to care for it after you do.

Your hair isn't broken — it's just asking you to handle it with a little more respect. And if you do, it'll carry you through until the new growth comes in strong.

# 5

# Physical Damage

## The Everyday Wear and Tear

Not all damage comes from a salon chair. A lot of it happens
slowly, every day, in the way you handle your hair. Tugging
with the wrong comb, throwing it in a tight ponytail, rubbing
it against a pillow — these little things add up. That's physical
damage. It's not one big event, it's death by a thousand cuts.

## What Physical Damage Looks Like

Imagine your hair strand as a piece of thread. Pull it too hard,
rub it against rough fabric, or tie it too tight — eventually it
frays, splits, and snaps. That's exactly what's happening when
you notice:

- **Breakage:** Little pieces of hair on your sink or shoulders.
- **Split Ends:** Strands unraveling at the tips like a rope.
- **Knots & Single-Strand Tangles:** Hair looping on itself

because the cuticle is roughed up.
- **Thinning in One Spot:** Constant tension from styles pulling the same area.
- **Frizz That Won't Smooth:** Damaged cuticles acting like Velcro.

## Everyday Habits That Cause It

Physical damage usually doesn't come from one mistake — it's repeated habits:

- **Brushing or combing too rough** (especially when dry or tangled).
- **Tight ponytails, braids, or buns** pulling on the hairline (traction alopecia).
- **Heat styling with no protection** (flat irons, blow-dryers).
- **Sleeping on cotton** — friction wears strands down overnight.
- **Over-manipulation** — touching, styling, or redoing hair too often.

Think of it like a favorite T-shirt. If you wash it every day, stretch the collar, and sleep in it, it's going to wear out faster.

## How to Manage and Prevent It

Damaged fabric doesn't mend itself, but you can protect it so it lasts longer. Hair works the same way.

- **Detangle with care.** Always detangle damp or with conditioner for slip. Start from the ends, work your way up.

Wide-tooth combs and your fingers are your best tools.

- **Loosen the tension.** Protective styles should protect — not strangle. If it feels tight on day one, it's too tight.
- **Protect your edges.** The hairline is fragile. Switch up partings, use satin scarves, and give your edges breaks.
- **Heat with caution.** If you use heat, keep it low to medium, never skip heat protectant, and don't pass the iron over the same spot five times.
- **Night care matters.** Satin pillowcase or bonnet. Cotton is like sandpaper — it steals moisture and causes friction.
- **Hands off.** The more you play with your hair, the more stress it goes through. Sometimes the best care is leaving it alone.

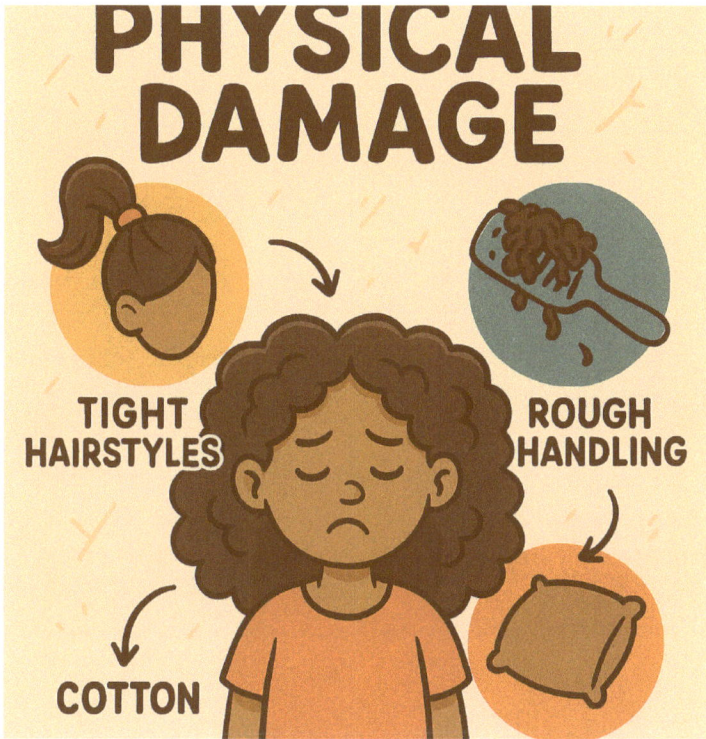

## Story From the Chair

A client once came in with thinning at the crown. She swore her products were failing her. But when I asked about her routine, she admitted: tight ponytail, every single day, for years. That tension had been slowly pulling on the same area until the hair said, "I'm done." We switched her up to looser buns, added satin scrunchies, and gave her scalp breaks. A few months later, new growth started coming in where the thinning had been.

29

## Takeaways

- Physical damage = everyday wear and tear.
- Rough handling, tension styles, heat, and friction are the main culprits.
- Split ends, breakage, thinning edges, and constant frizz are the warning signs.
- Be gentle, reduce tension, protect at night, and trim when needed.
- Healthy hair isn't just about what you put *on* it — it's about how you *treat* it.

☞ If chemical damage is like spilling bleach on your favorite jeans, physical damage is like wearing them out until they tear. In both cases, prevention and protection are your best tools.

# 6

# Weather Vs. Your Hair

## The Humidity Factor

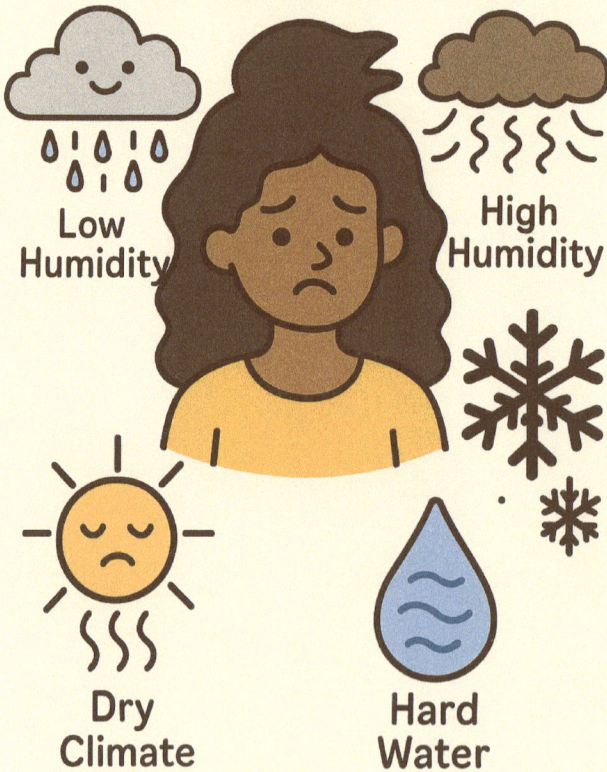

Ever notice how your hair has a whole personality shift depending on the weather? In the summer, it's puffing up like a cloud. In the winter, it's dry and snapping. That's not bad products — that's the air around you. Weather is one of the biggest "invisible products" your hair deals with every day.

## Low Humidity — The Desert Effect

When the air is dry, it's like living in a desert. Your humectants (like glycerin or aloe) try to pull moisture in, but there's nothing in the air to grab. So instead, they pull it *out of your hair*. That's why your strands feel brittle and thirsty.

**Fix it:**

- Load up on moisture on wash day.
- Seal it in with heavier oils and butters.
- Rock protective styles so your ends don't dry out.

**Analogy:** Dry air is like winter lips. If you don't lock in that chapstick, you'll be cracking all day.

## High Humidity — The Frizz Factory

On the flip side, when the air is full of water (think Miami in July), humectants pull in *too much* moisture. Your strands swell up like a sponge and frizz takes over.

**Fix it:**

- Use gels, mousses, or products with strong film-formers to keep the cuticle flat.
- Seal lightly with oils like jojoba or grapeseed.
- Look for "anti-humidity" or "frizz-control" on the label.

**Analogy:** High humidity is like eating too much at a buffet. Too much of a good thing makes you uncomfortable.

## Cold Weather — The Silent Thief

Winter air outside + heaters inside = double dryness. That's when you start getting static, brittle ends, and that "hair breaking under your beanie" feeling.
  **Fix it:**

- Swap in creams and butters for heavier protection.
- Deep condition weekly.
- Wear satin-lined hats or wrap your hair before going out.

**Analogy:** Winter is like leaving food uncovered in the fridge. It dries out faster than you think.

## Hard Water & Chlorine — The Sneaky Saboteurs

Not weather, but still environmental. Hard water leaves a chalky film on your strands. Chlorine strips oils and leaves your hair dry.
  **Fix it:**

- Use a chelating or clarifying shampoo once a month.
- Rinse hair with clean water before swimming so it doesn't soak up chlorine.
- Deep condition after pool days.

## Story From the Chair

I had two clients use the same leave-in. One lived in Arizona, the other in Miami. Arizona said, "This stuff makes my hair crunchy and stiff." Miami said, "This stuff makes my hair puff up like cotton candy." Same product, totally different outcome. Why? The air. Once we adjusted — butters for Arizona, gel for Miami — both of them loved that same leave-in.

## Takeaways

- Dry climate = seal with butters/oils.
- Humid climate = lock down with gels/foams.
- Cold weather = protect with creams and satin.
- Hard water = clarify/chelating.
- Swimming = rinse first, condition after.

Weather is the product you can't buy, but it's the one you always have to work with. Learn how to play the game, and your hair will win every season.

# 7

# Common Hair Problems & Fixes

Even with the best routine, problems can pop up. Think of it like gardening: sometimes the soil dries out, pests show up, or plants shed their leaves. None of it means the garden is ruined — it just needs the right care. Here are the most common hair struggles and how to handle them.

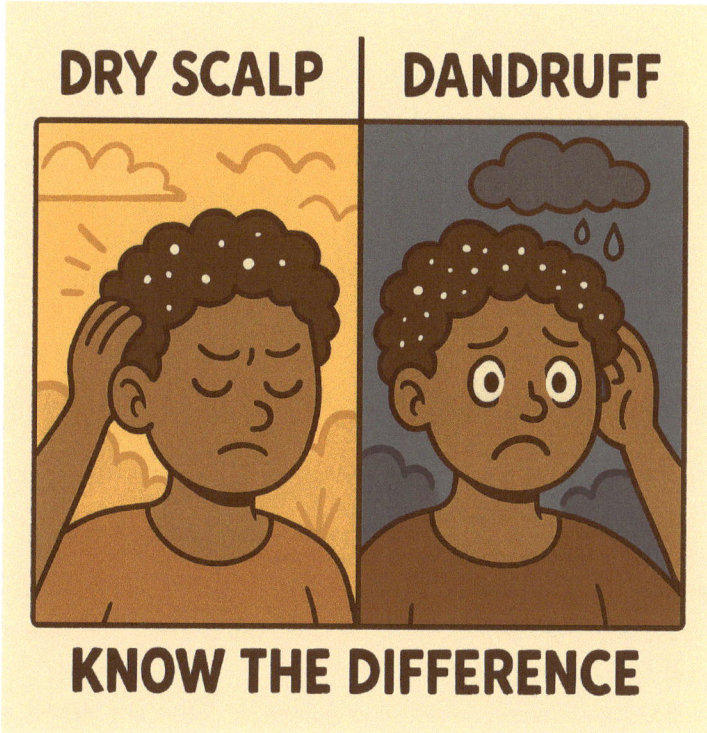

## Dandruff vs. Dry Scalp — Snowflakes or Storm?

Flakes on your shoulders can mean two different things:

- **Dry scalp:** Tiny, white, dusty flakes. Your scalp feels tight or itchy.
- **Dandruff:** Bigger, oily flakes that stick to the scalp. Often itchy, sometimes with redness.

**Fix:**

- Dry scalp → Use a moisturizing shampoo and light oil on the scalp.
- Dandruff → Wash regularly with a dandruff shampoo and avoid heavy oils that trap yeast.

**Story:** One client kept piling oil onto her scalp, thinking it would fix her flakes. But it was dandruff, not dryness. Once she switched to a medicated shampoo and lightened up on the oils, her flakes disappeared.

## Chronically Dry Hair — Thirsty Strands

Dry hair is like soil that never holds water. It feels rough, looks dull, and breaks easily.

**Causes:** Over-washing, harsh shampoos, skipping conditioner, or not sealing moisture.

**Fix:** Moisturize consistently, seal with oil, and deep condition weekly.

**Tip:** If your hair drinks product but feels dry again by morning, you may have high-porosity hair. Layer moisture and seal properly.

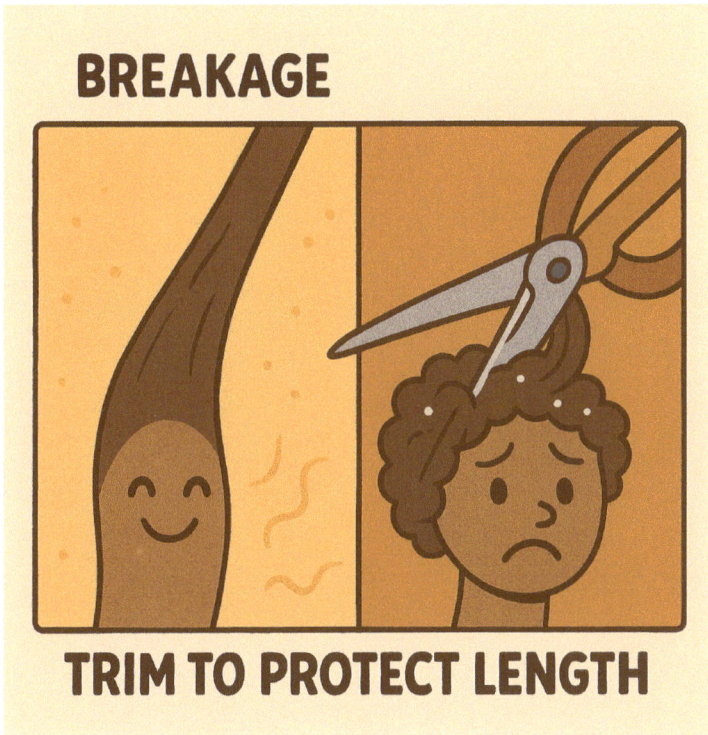

## Breakage and Split Ends — Cracked Glass

Split ends are like cracks in a windshield. If you don't fix them, they spread upward. Breakage is when strands snap before they should.

**Causes:** Heat, chemicals, rough handling, or skipped trims.

**Fix:** Trim regularly, use protective styles, and handle hair gently.

**Trick:** If your ends tangle easily or feel rough even after conditioning, it's time for a trim.

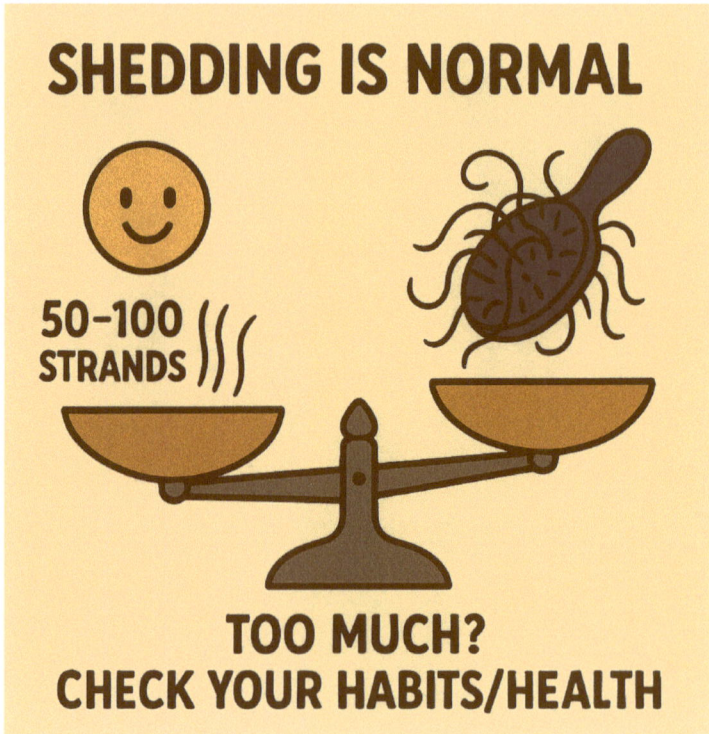

## Excessive Shedding — Falling Leaves

Everyone sheds hair daily — it's part of the growth cycle. But if you're losing more than usual for weeks at a time, it's worth paying attention.

**Causes:** Stress, diet changes, tight hairstyles, postpartum changes, or medical issues.

**Fix:** Loosen up styles, eat balanced meals, manage stress, and consult a doctor if shedding doesn't slow down.

**Story:** A client once panicked about "going bald" after having her baby. It was postpartum shedding — completely normal. I reassured her, and within months her hair filled back in.

## Traction Alopecia — Pulled-Out Edges

Edges are fragile. Constant tight braids, ponytails, or slick-backs can pull them right out.

**Signs:** Thinning hairline, sore bumps, shiny smooth patches.

**Fix:** Stop the tension. Rotate styles, give your scalp rest, and massage gently to stimulate growth.

**Truth:** Once follicles are scarred, hair may not grow back. Prevention is key.

## Knots and Tangles — Nature's Velcro

Curls and coils love each other so much they sometimes tie themselves together. That's how you get single-strand knots or tangles.

**Fix:**

- Detangle with slip (conditioner or leave-in).
- Stretch hair at night (twists, braids, or pineappling).
- Trim regularly to prevent split ends from knotting.

**Trick:** A little patience saves a lot of hair. Forcing a knot always costs you length.

## Takeaways

- Flakes aren't all the same — know the difference between dandruff and dryness.
- Dry hair needs moisture, sealing, and consistent care.
- Split ends must be trimmed — there's no product that glues them backvisua.
- Shedding is normal, but sudden excess can signal stress or health issues.
- Edges need protection — tension styles cause traction alopecia.
- Knots and tangles need patience and prevention, not force.

# 8

# Porosity

## How Your Hair Drinks Water

Porosity is one of those words that sounds scientific, but all it really means is: **how well your hair drinks and holds onto water.** Think of each strand as a fabric. Some fabrics resist water, some soak it up, and some absorb but never hold onto it. That's why the same product can give one person silky curls and another person dry frizz. It all comes down to how "thirsty" your hair is — and how long it stays quenched.

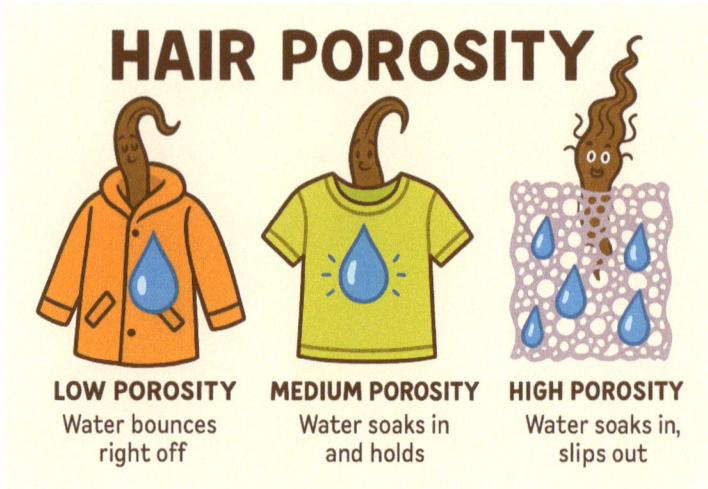

## Low Porosity — The Raincoat

Low-porosity hair has cuticles that lay flat and tight, like shingles on a roof or a raincoat. Water just beads up and slides off.

- **What it's like:** Your hair takes forever to get wet, products sit on top, and heavy creams leave a greasy film instead of softness.
- **The fix:**
- Add heat or steam when deep conditioning to "open" the cuticle.
- Use lighter products — milks, sprays, and liquid-based leave-ins.
- Clarify regularly to avoid buildup, since nothing penetrates

easily.

**Analogy:** Imagine trying to water a plant with waxy leaves —
the water slides right off. You need to soften the surface before
it can drink.

## Medium Porosity — The Cotton T-Shirt

Medium-porosity hair is the easiest to manage. The cuticle isn't
too tight or too open — it lets moisture in and holds it well. It's
like a cotton shirt: it soaks water, but doesn't cling to it forever.

- **What it's like:** Products absorb easily, hair feels manage-
  able, styles last, and moisture doesn't vanish right away.
- **The fix:**
- Just maintain balance.
- Alternate between moisture masks and light protein.
- Don't overload with heavy butters if you don't need them.

**Analogy:** Medium porosity is like Goldilocks' porridge — not
too much, not too little, just right.

## High Porosity — The Lace Fabric

High-porosity hair has holes in the cuticle — either naturally
or from damage (bleach, heat, dye). Moisture rushes in fast,
but leaks right back out. It's like lace fabric — water soaks it
instantly, but it can't hold onto it.

- **What it's like:** Hair dries super fast after washing, tangles
  easily, frizzes in humidity, and always feels thirsty.

- **The fix:**
- Layer products (LOC or LCO) so moisture has backup guards.
- Use heavier sealants (castor oil, shea butter) to "plug the holes."
- Protein treatments patch weak spots in the cuticle.

**Analogy:** High porosity is like carrying water in a strainer — it fills up, but it won't stay unless you patch the holes or cover the top.

## How to Tell Which You Have

Forget the cup test (dropping hair in water isn't reliable). Pay attention to how your hair acts:

- Takes forever to get wet + buildup? **Low.**
- Responds to most products + pretty easy to manage? **Medium.**
- Dries super fast + frizzes or tangles? **High.**

## Story From the Chair

Two clients sat in my chair on the same day.

- The first had **low-porosity coils.** She complained her conditioners "never worked." Once I put her under steam with the same conditioner, her hair soaked it up like a sponge.
- The second had **high-porosity curls from bleaching.** She said her hair was "always thirsty." We layered leave-in, cream, and oil, and for the first time, her hair stayed soft

for more than 24 hours.

Both said the same thing: *"My hair is dry."* The difference was porosity.

## Takeaways

- **Low porosity = raincoat.** Hard to get moisture in → use heat, lighter products, and clarify.
- **Medium porosity = cotton.** Holds moisture well → just balance protein and hydration.
- **High porosity = lace.** Moisture slips out → seal with oils/butters and use protein to patch.

Once you understand porosity, you stop playing guessing games with your products. It's like knowing whether your fabric is silk, cotton, or lace — you'll wash, treat, and care for it differently, and it'll last longer.

# 9

# Hair Care Methods

## Finding Your Formula

There's no magic product that works for everyone — what really matters is the **method** you use. Methods are like recipes: the same ingredients can give you totally different results depending on how you combine them. The trick is finding the recipe your hair responds to best.

Just like the petals of a flower, your hair strands should be protected from damage.

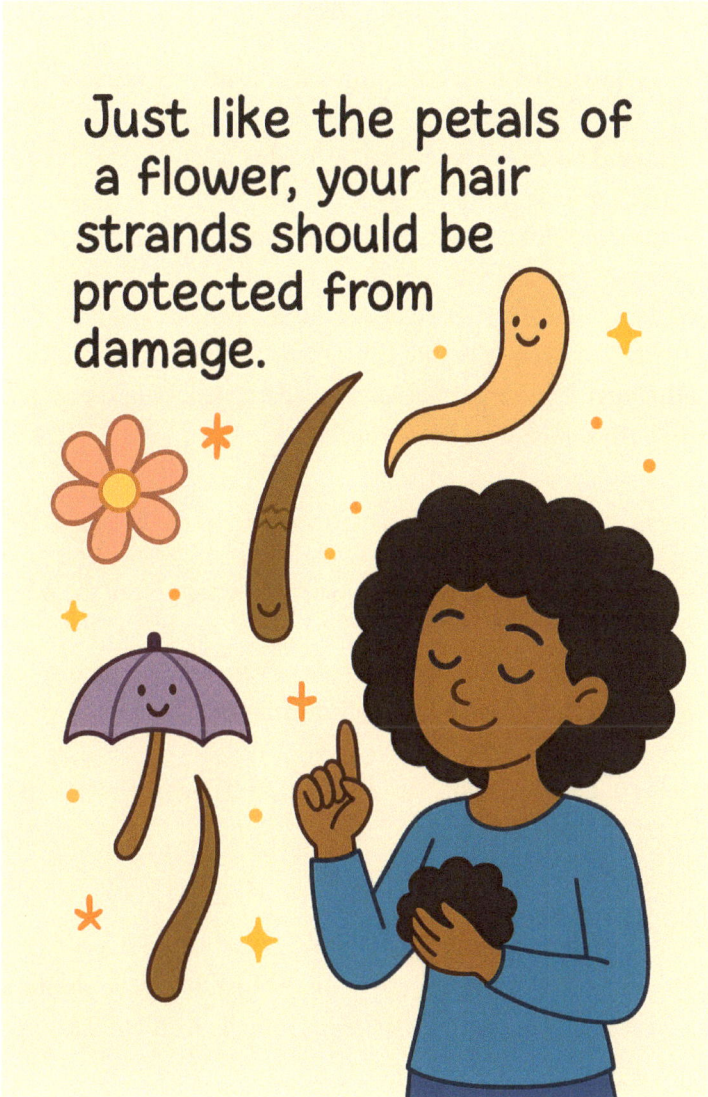

## The LOC Method (Liquid–Oil–Cream)

This is the OG natural hair routine. It's all about layers.

- **Liquid (water or leave-in):** Hydrates.
- **Oil:** Locks it in.
- **Cream:** Adds richness and definition.

Best for: Thick, high-porosity hair that dries out easily.
Watch out: Too heavy for fine or low-porosity hair.
**Analogy:** It's like putting lotion on damp skin, then sealing it with butter. Moisture stays trapped.

## The LCO Method (Liquid–Cream–Oil)

Same idea as LOC, but flipped. The cream goes before the oil.

- Great for low-porosity hair that rejects heavy layering.
- Gives softness without weighing hair down.

**Analogy:** Like cooking pasta — water first, then sauce, then a drizzle of olive oil.

## The Baggy Method

This one's like putting your hair in a sauna. You apply a moisturizer, cover with a plastic cap, and let heat build up.

- Helps moisture penetrate deeper.
- Works wonders for dry ends.

**Analogy:** Like steaming vegetables so they soak up flavor instead of boiling them dry.

## The Greenhouse Effect

Similar to baggy, but focused on oils. You oil your hair, cover it, and let your body heat create a humid "greenhouse" overnight.

- Boosts softness and elasticity.
- Can help with length retention.

**Analogy:** Like putting a plant in a greenhouse — it thrives in warmth and humidity.

## The Inversion Method

Warm oil scalp massage + flipping your head upside down for a few minutes.

- Increases blood flow to follicles.
- Sometimes used as a growth hack.

**Analogy:** Like watering a plant and then putting it closer to the sun — you're feeding the roots.

## Co-Washing (Conditioner-Only Washing)

Skip shampoo, use conditioner to cleanse.

- Keeps moisture in.
- Perfect for curls that hate frequent shampooing.

· But: Can cause buildup if you never clarify.

**Analogy:** Like washing your face with a gentle cleanser instead of harsh soap.

## Max Hydration Method

This is the bootcamp routine. It's multi-step: clarify, deep condition, clay rinse, leave-in, and gel — often repeated for days in a row.

· Gives definition and moisture to tight curls and coils.
· Time-consuming, but results can be dramatic.

**Analogy:** Like sending your hair on a spa retreat. It comes back refreshed, but it's a lot of work.

## Ayurvedic Methods

Rooted in Indian tradition, using herbs like amla, henna, fenu-greek, bhringraj.

· Strengthens, thickens, and boosts scalp health.
· Works slow and steady, but powerful over time.

**Analogy:** Like replacing energy drinks with herbal teas. Results are gentler, but longer lasting.

## The LOC vs. LCO Debate

Here's the funny thing: people argue all day about which one is "right." The truth? Both work — it depends on your hair.

- High-porosity hair: LOC usually wins.
- Low-porosity hair: LCO keeps it lighter.

**Moral:** Don't marry one method. Try both.

## Other Methods People Don't Always Name

**Pre-Poo (Pre-Shampoo Treatment):**

- Oil, conditioner, or aloe applied *before* shampooing to protect from dryness.
- *Analogy:* Like marinating meat before cooking so it doesn't dry out.

**Rice Water Rinse:**

- Fermented rice water used to strengthen with amino acids.
- *Analogy:* Like giving your hair a protein smoothie.

**Clay Wash (Rhassoul/Bentonite):**

- Natural clays pull out dirt and product buildup while adding minerals.
- *Analogy:* Like using a detox face mask, but for your strands.

**Tea Rinses:**

- Black tea, green tea, or herbal teas poured over hair. Can reduce shedding and add shine.
- *Analogy:* Like giving your hair a vitamin boost.

**Scalp Oiling & Massages:**

- Oils with peppermint, rosemary, or castor massaged into the scalp.
- *Analogy:* Like a workout warm-up for your roots — blood flow = growth support.

## Story From the Chair

I had one client who kept switching products every two weeks, frustrated that "nothing works." When I asked how she was using them, she admitted she just slapped them on randomly. I taught her the LOC method — suddenly, those same products actually worked. Another client was struggling with dryness no matter what she did. We tried the Greenhouse Effect on her ends. Two weeks later she came back, shocked, saying, "My hair finally feels soft in the morning." Same products, different method — game changer.

## Quick Takeaways

- Methods matter more than brands.
- LOC and LCO = moisture layering (test which works for you).
- Baggy & Greenhouse = deep moisture hacks.
- Inversion = growth stimulation.
- Co-Wash = gentle cleanse, but clarify sometimes.
- Max Hydration = intense curl spa.

- Ayurvedic & herbal = holistic, slow build.
- Pre-poo, clay, rice water, and tea rinses are bonus tools.

Think of methods like recipes. The ingredients (products) don't change much — but the order, timing, and technique can make or break your results.

# 10

# Products & Ingredients

Walking down the hair care aisle can feel like walking into a jungle. Bright bottles shouting promises, words you can't pronounce, and prices all over the place. But here's the truth: the right products aren't always the fanciest ones. It's about knowing what each type does and how it fits your routine.

## Start With the Core Four

1. **Shampoo** — clears the scalp so follicles can breathe.
2. **Conditioner** — softens, adds slip, reduces breakage.
3. **Leave-in** — lightweight moisture that stays put.
4. **Oil/Butter** — **seals** moisture in (doesn't create it).

**Rule:** Master these first. Stylers (gels, foams, creams, edge control) are optional add-ons.

# Products & Ingredients

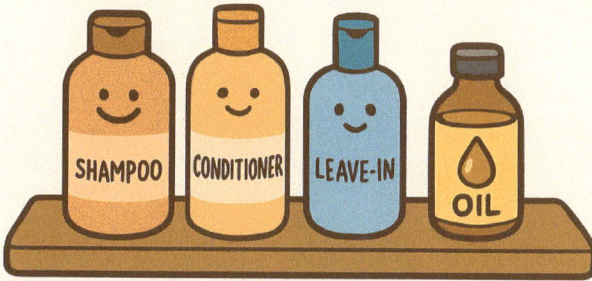

## Shampoos
- Moisturizing
- Clarifying
- Protein/Anti-breakage

## Conditioners
- Rinse-out
- Deep
- Leave-in

## Oils
- Sealing • Butter • Essential

## Ingredients to Watch

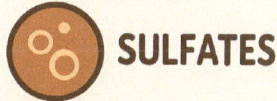 **SULFATES**

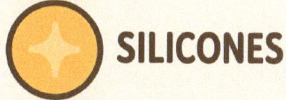 **SILICONES**

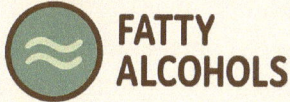 **FATTY ALCOHOLS**

©

## Shampoos — The Clean-Up Crew

Shampoos are like different kinds of soap for your hair. Some are gentle, some are deep cleaners, and some add extra benefits. Think of shampoo as the reset button. Its job is to lift dirt, sweat, oil, and product buildup from your scalp and hair. But how it does that makes all the difference.

**Moisturizing Shampoo:** Gentle wash for regular use. Cleans without leaving hair squeaky-dry.
  *Best for*: Dry or curly hair.
  *Analogy:* Like washing your face with a creamy cleanser instead of bar soap.

**Clarifying Shampoo:** A deep reset for heavy buildup, sweat, or chlorine. Think of it as a detox — but only once in a while (monthly or after swimming).
  *Best for*: Occasional use (1–2x/month).
  *Analogy:* Like spring cleaning your house — you don't do it every day, but when you

**Protein/Anti-Breakage Shampoo:** Adds light strength on wash day. Works for hair that feels weak. Infused with keratin, silk, or wheat proteins to strengthen weak strands.
  *Best for*: Chemically treated or damaged hair.
  *Analogy:* Like adding reinforcement beams to a shaky bridge.

**Volumizing Shampoo:** Gives fine or flat hair some lift. Light on the strands so they don't get weighed down. Lightweight, adds body without weighing hair down.
  *Best for*: Fine or limp hair.

*Analogy:* Like fluffing up a pillow.

**Tip:** You don't need ten shampoos. Pick one everyday shampoo, and keep a clarifying one for those "reset" days.

**Story:** I had a client who used clarifying shampoo every week because she liked the "squeaky clean" feel. Her hair was dry and brittle. Once she switched to a moisturizing shampoo and saved clarifying for once a month, her hair softened up within weeks.

## Conditioners — The Repair Crew

Conditioner is non-negotiable. It restores balance after washing and makes detangling easier. If shampoo strips away the dirt, conditioner swoops in to restore balance. It smooths the cuticle, adds softness, and makes hair easier to manage.

**Rinse-Out Conditioner:** Quick hydration and slip after shampoo. The everyday softener. Quick moisture, easy slip.
*Analogy:* Like putting lotion on after washing your hands.

**Deep Conditioner/Mask:** Richer treatment that stays on longer. Great weekly or biweekly. Thick, heavy-duty formulas that penetrate deeper. Usually left on 15–30 minutes.
*Analogy:* Like a spa day for your hair — not every day, but a big difference when you do.

## Leave-In Conditioner

Lightweight hydration that stays in your hair. Helps with frizz, dryness, and everyday manageability.

*Analogy:* Like carrying lip balm in your pocket — protection on the go.

**Trick:** If your hair feels rough after a wash, you skipped conditioner — go back and fix it.

## What a Leave-In Really Does

Leave-ins aren't just "extra conditioner." They're lighter, designed to stay on the hair without weighing it down or making it greasy. Their job is:

- **Hydration:** Adds moisture between wash days.
- **Slip:** Makes detangling easier.
- **Protection:** Guards hair from heat, UV rays, and pollution.
- **Styling Base:** Preps curls, coils, or straight strands for whatever comes next.

**Analogy:** If shampoo is the shower and rinse-out conditioner is lotion, then leave-in is chapstick — always on hand, always there to keep you from cracking.

## Who Needs a Leave-In?

- **Curly/Coily Hair:** Absolutely. It fights dryness and defines curls.
- **Color-Treated Hair:** Extra hydration + protection from fading.

- **Fine Hair:** Yes — just choose a lightweight spray instead of a cream.
- **Straight Hair:** Not mandatory, but great if you use heat or live in dry climates.

Basically? If your hair sees the sun, heat tools, or even just city air — you need a leave-in.

## Types of Leave-In Conditioners

**Sprays (Lightweight)**

- Best for fine or low-porosity hair.
- Mist absorbs easily without heaviness.
- *Analogy:* Like carrying a water bottle in your bag — quick refresh anytime.

**Lotions/Milks (Medium Weight)**

- Great for normal or wavy/curly hair.
- Balanced hydration + definition.
- *Analogy:* Like a daily moisturizer for your skin.

**Creams/Butters (Heavy)**

- Best for thick, coarse, or high-porosity hair.
- Provides lasting moisture and curl clumping.
- *Analogy:* Like shea butter on ashy skin — rich and lasting.

## Story From the Chair

One of my clients said, "My hair always feels amazing on wash day but turns crunchy two days later." When I asked if she used a leave-in, she shook her head. We added a spray leave-in to her mid-week routine. Next visit? She said, "It feels soft all week now." The difference wasn't in her shampoo or conditioner — it was that daily bodyguard, the leave-in.

## Why They Work Best Together

Shampoo without conditioner is like washing dishes without drying them — clean, but not finished. Conditioner seals the cuticle that shampoo opens, locking in moisture and protecting strands from frizz and breakage.

And conditioner without shampoo? That's like putting perfume on without showering — you're masking buildup, not removing it.

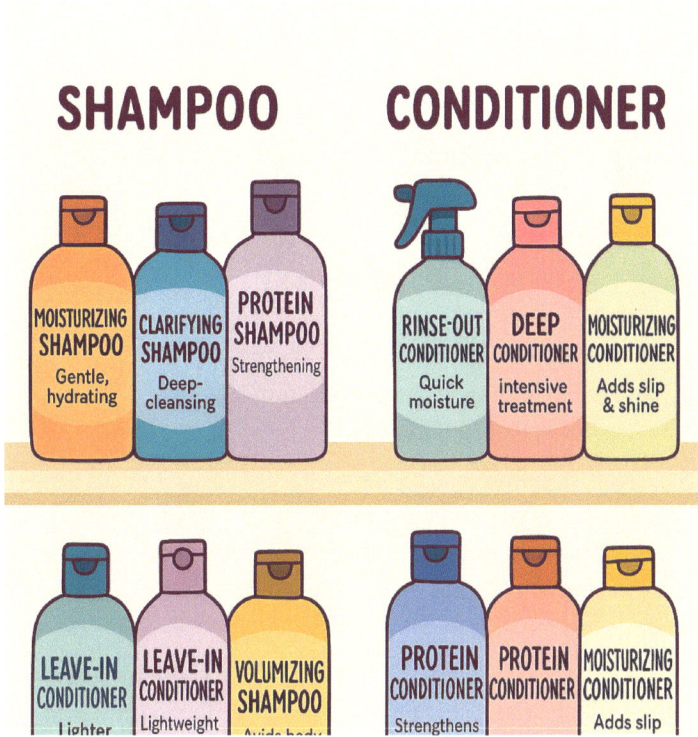

## SHAMPOO

**MOISTURIZING SHAMPOO** — Gentle, hydrating

**CLARIFYING SHAMPOO** — Deep-cleansing

**PROTEIN SHAMPOO** — Strengthening

**LEAVE-IN CONDITIONER** — Lighter

**LEAVE-IN CONDITIONER** — Lightweight

**VOLUMIZING SHAMPOO** — Adds body

## CONDITIONER

**RINSE-OUT CONDITIONER** — Quick moisture

**DEEP CONDITIONER** — intensive treatment

**MOISTURIZING CONDITIONER** — Adds slip & shine

**PROTEIN CONDITIONER** — Strengthens

**PROTEIN CONDITIONER**

**MOISTURIZING CONDITIONER** — Adds slip

## Oils and Butters — The Sealers

Oils and butters don't moisturize by themselves — they lock in the moisture you already added.

- **Moisturizing Oils (sink in a little):** Olive, avocado, coconut.
- **Sealing Oils (sit on top):** Castor, jojoba, grapeseed.
- **Butters:** Shea, mango, cocoa. Great for thick or high-porosity hair, but heavy for fine textures.

63

· **Essential Oils:** Peppermint, tea tree, rosemary — use sparingly and always mix with a carrier oil.

**Tip:** If your scalp is itchy after using oils, you're using too much. A few drops go a long way.

## Stylers — What They Actually Do

· **Gels (holds shape):** look for film-formers (PVP, acrylates) or naturals (flax/sea moss gels). Apply to **wet** hair; let a cast form, then **scrunch out the crunch** once dry.
· **Creams/Custards (soft hold + moisture):** define twists/braids; great for thicker textures or high porosity.
· **Foams/Mousses (lightweight lift):** great for fine hair or roller/rod sets; look for **polyquaterniums** for frizz control without weight.
· **Edge control:** occasional use; cleanse edges well to avoid buildup.

**Layering 101:** try **LCO** (Leave-in → Cream → Oil) or **LOC** (Leave-in → Oil → Cream). High porosity often loves LOC; low porosity usually prefers lighter LCO or just Leave-in + a few drops of oil.

## Preservatives — The Unsung Heroes

No one likes to think about preservatives, but without them, your favorite conditioner would spoil like milk.

· **Tip:** Don't fear preservatives. They keep your products safe.

The key is to notice if your scalp reacts to specific ones and switch if needed.

## Ingredients — The Fine Print

Reading the back of a bottle can feel like reading another language, but here's what matters most:

### Sulfates — The Strong Soap

Sulfates are heavy-duty cleansers. They're like dish soap: they cut grease fast but can leave things squeaky-dry.

- **Good for:** Clearing heavy buildup, chlorine, or product overload.
- **Risk:** Can strip natural oils if used too often.
- **Tip:** If you use lots of gels, edge control, or butters, a sulfate shampoo every now and then is your reset button.

**Story:** A client once told me her curls were always dry. She used a sulfate shampoo every wash day. Once she switched to a gentle cleanser and used sulfate only once a month, her curls held moisture again.

### Silicones — The Smooth Talkers

Silicones coat your hair, making it feel silky and look shiny. They're like putting wax on a car — great shine, but buildup if you don't wash it off.

- **Good for:** Protecting hair from heat, adding slip, controlling frizz.
- **Risk:** Can weigh down fine hair or block moisture if not washed out.
- **Tip:** If you use silicones, pair them with an occasional clarifying wash to reset.

## Alcohols — Not All Created Equal

When people hear "alcohol," they think instant dryness. But there are two kinds:

- **Bad alcohols (drying):** Isopropyl alcohol, ethanol. These evaporate fast and strip moisture.
- **Good alcohols (fatty, moisturizing):** Cetyl, stearyl, cetearyl. These actually soften and condition hair.

**Trick:** Don't fear all alcohols. If you see cetyl or stearyl on the label, it's actually a good thing.

## Fragrance — The Sneaky Irritant

Fragrance makes products smell amazing, but it can be harsh on sensitive scalps.

- **Good for:** A pleasant experience.
- **Risk:** Itchiness or irritation for some people.
- **Tip:** If your scalp is acting up, try a fragrance-free product.

**Story:** A client once told me her "new miracle product" made her scalp burn. When we checked the label, the first ingredient was alcohol. Switching to a gentler, fragrance-free option solved the problem instantly.

## Choosing the Right Combo

- Dry hair? Moisturizing shampoo + moisturizing conditioner.
- Oily scalp with buildup? Clarifying shampoo + light conditioner.
- Weak, limp curls? Protein shampoo + moisturizing deep conditioner.
- Fine hair? Volumizing shampoo + light leave-in.

**Trick:** Don't buy based on hype. Buy based on what your hair needs *that week.*

## How to Choose Products Without Stress

1. **Know your hair type:** Porosity, density, and elasticity guide what products you need.
2. **Keep it simple:** A good shampoo, a conditioner, a leave-in, an oil. That's your starter pack.
3. **Watch how your hair reacts:** If it feels dry, rough, or heavy, the product isn't right for you.
4. **Don't chase trends:** Just because it's viral doesn't mean it's for your head.

**Pro Tip:** Your hair will always tell you the truth. Listen to it more than the label.

## Takeaways

- Shampoo = clean. Conditioner = restore.
- Moisturizing, clarifying, protein, volumizing shampoos all serve different purposes.
- Rinse-out, leave-in, deep, protein, and moisturizing conditioners each have their place.
- Leave-in = hydration, protection, styling support all in one.
- Sprays = light. Lotions = balanced. Creams = heavy-duty.
- Always apply to damp hair, focusing on ends.
- Great for curls, coils, color-treated, dry, or heat-styled hair.
- Think of it as the "insurance policy" for your wash day.
- The right pair depends on your hair's current state — not just what's trending.
- Oils and butters lock in moisture, they don't create it.
- Labels matter, but results matter more.
- Build a simple kit that matches your hair type and lifestyle.

# 11

# Decoding Like a Pro

## Cracking the Label Code

Walking down the hair care aisle can feel like walking through a loud marketplace. Every bottle is yelling:

- *"Ultra-Mega Moisture!"*
- *"Extreme Strength!"*
- *"Miracle Growth in 7 Days!"*

The truth? Most of those words are just marketing. The real story isn't in the front label — it's in the **ingredient list** on the back. Once you know how to read it, you'll see through the hype like a pro.

# HOW TO READ A LABEL

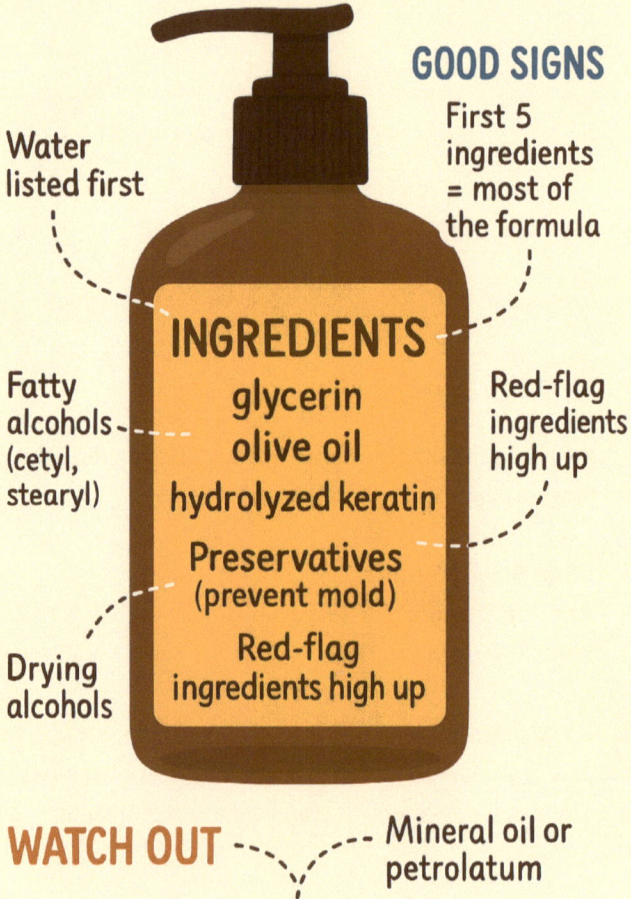

**GOOD SIGNS**

First 5
ingredients
= most of
the formula

Water
listed first

## INGREDIENTS

glycerin
olive oil
hydrolyzed keratin

Preservatives
(prevent mold)

Red-flag
ingredients high up

Fatty
alcohols
(cetyl,
stearyl)

Red-flag
ingredients
high up

Drying
alcohols

**WATCH OUT**

Mineral oil or
petrolatum

## The First Five Rule — Meet the Main Cast

Think of the ingredient list like a TV show. The **first five ingredients** are the main actors — they carry the whole plot. Everyone else is just background noise.

- If water is first, that's a good sign. Real hydration starts here.
- If a drying alcohol or heavy grease is up top, expect dryness or weight, no matter what the front says.
- If "exotic oils" are tucked at the very end? That's just decoration. There's barely any in there.

**Quick Tip:** Flip the bottle and read the cast list before you buy the hype.

# THE THREE MUSKETERS
## *of* Moisture

**Humectant → Emollient → Occlusive**
adds water        smooths          locks
                  and softens      moisture in

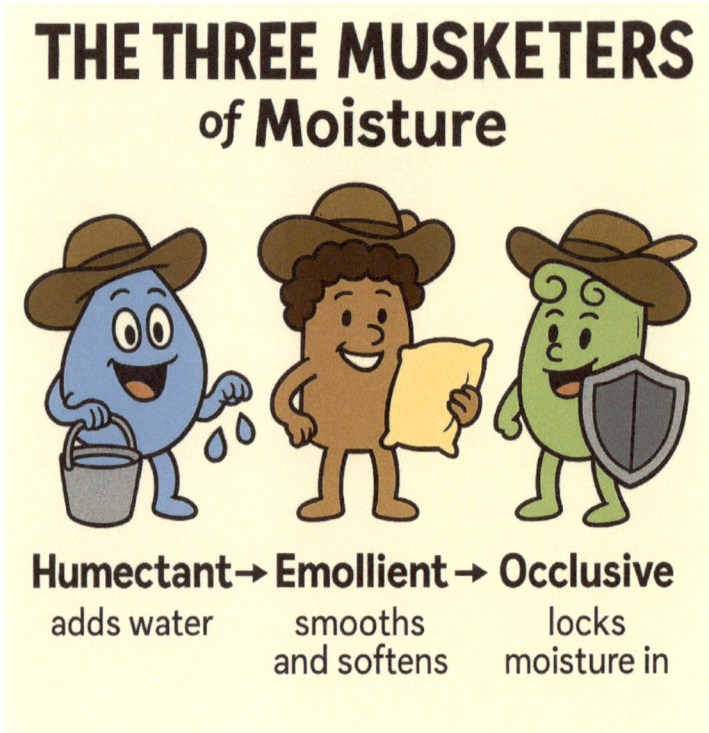

## Humectants, Emollients, Occlusives — The Dream Team

Your hair needs three types of players working together:

- Humectants (like glycerin, aloe, honey) → pull in water. Think of them like the water in your recipe.
- Emollients (like olive oil, shea butter, esters) → soften, smooth, and add slip. That's your seasoning.

- Occlusives (like castor oil, silicones, beeswax) → lock it all in. That's the lid on the pot.

No water + only a lid = dry meal. Same with hair — sealing dry hair just locks in dryness.

## Protein — The Patch Kit

Proteins are like patching up a hole in your favorite jeans. They don't make the fabric brand new, but they fill in weak spots so it holds together longer.

- Look for "hydrolyzed" proteins — those are small enough to actually stick to your hair.
- Mushy, weak hair that won't hold a style? Protein helps.
- Stiff, straw-like hair? That's protein overload. Step back and balance with moisture.

## Alcohols — The Cousins at the Cookout

Not all alcohols are the same.

- Bad alcohols: isopropyl, ethanol, SD alcohol. These evaporate quick and dry your hair out.
- Good alcohols: cetyl, cetearyl, stearyl. These are creamy thickeners that actually moisturize.

So don't panic when you see "alcohol."

## Silicones — The Shiny Coat

Silicones are like makeup for your hair.

- They smooth frizz, add shine, protect against heat.
- Some build up (dimethicone, cyclomethicone). You'll need a clarifying wash sometimes.
- Others rinse right out (PEG-modified silicones).

Nothing wrong with them — just don't forget to "wash your face" (aka clarify).

## Fragrance & Preservatives — The Extras

Fragrance makes your product smell good, but if your scalp is sensitive, it can be the hidden reason you're itchy.

Preservatives keep your product from molding. Don't be scared of them — you don't want your conditioner turning into a science project.

## Red Flags to Watch For

- Mineral oil or petrolatum as the first few ingredients (unless you're purposely sealing).
- Drying alcohols up top.
- Protein overload when your hair doesn't need it.
- Fancy oils at the very end → marketing sprinkles.

## The Quick-Skim Method

Next time you're in the aisle, ask yourself 3 things:

- Is water in the first three?
- Do I see a humectant, emollient, or protein depending on my need?
- Any red flags near the top?

If it passes all three, it's probably worth a shot.

## Story from the Chair

A client once bragged about her new "argan oil conditioner." She flipped the bottle — argan oil was almost the last ingredient. What was really in it? Water, glycerin, and cetearyl alcohol. That's what made her hair soft, not the argan.

She looked at me and said, "So I just paid extra for a sprinkle of argan?"

Yup. That's marketing for you.

## Takeaways

- The first five ingredients tell the truth.
- Humectants = water, Emollients = softness, Occlusives = seal.
- Proteins patch weak spots but need balance.
- Alcohols aren't all bad — some are your friends.
- Silicones smooth and protect but need clarifying.
- Preservatives are protection, fragrance can be a trigger.

Once you learn to decode labels, you'll never be fooled by shiny marketing again. You'll buy what actually works — and your hair will thank you.

# 12

# Oils and Butters

Oils and Butters — Locking It All In

# Oils & Butters

**Moisturizing Oils**

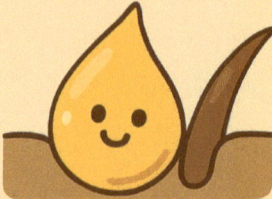

Olive/Avocado/Coconut

**Sealing Oils**

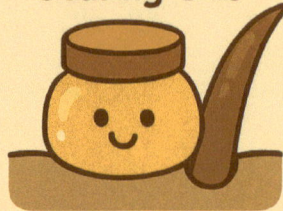

Sealing oils lock moisture in.

**Essential Oils**

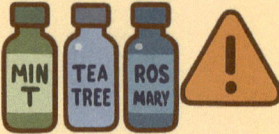

MINT  TEA TREE  ROSMARY

Strong — always dilute

**Butters**

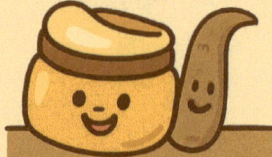

Butters protect— heavy but powerful

## Seal it or lose it

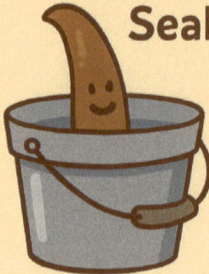

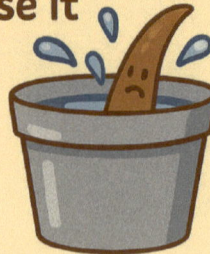

Oils and butters are like the finishing touch to your routine. They don't replace moisture, but they *trap it in*, keeping your hair soft and protected. Think of them as the lid on a water bottle — without it, everything leaks out.

## Moisturizing Oils — The Soakers

These oils can actually sink into the strand a little, adding softness and shine.

- **Examples:** Coconut, olive, avocado.
- **Best for:** Hair that feels rough or dry.
- **Tip:** Warm a small amount in your hands and smooth it over damp hair. Don't pour it on — a few drops go a long way.

**Story:** A client used to drench her curls in coconut oil daily. Her hair felt greasy but still dry. Once we cut it back to a few drops on damp hair, her curls stayed soft without being weighed down.

## Sealing Oils — The Guards

Sealing oils don't go inside the strand — they sit on top and lock moisture in.

- **Examples:** Castor, jojoba, grapeseed.
- **Best for:** High-porosity hair that loses water fast.
- **Tip:** Apply after leave-in conditioner or cream. Always "seal" in the moisture, don't just oil dry hair.

**Trick:** Castor oil is heavy — use sparingly, especially on fine hair.

## Butters — The Heavy Protectors

Butters are thick and rich, like a winter coat for your hair.

- **Examples:** Shea butter, mango butter, cocoa butter.
- **Best for:** Thick, coily, or high-porosity hair.
- **Avoid:** Using too much on fine or low-porosity hair — it can feel waxy.

**Tip:** Melt shea butter between your palms before applying for a smoother finish.

## Essential Oils — The Boosters

Essential oils are strong, concentrated oils that need to be diluted. Think of them like spices — a little adds flavor, too much ruins the dish.

- **Examples:**
- Peppermint — stimulates scalp and blood flow.
- Tea tree — soothes itch and reduces dandruff.
- Rosemary — supports growth and circulation.
- **Use:** Mix a few drops into a carrier oil (like olive or jojoba). Never apply directly to the scalp.

**Story:** A client once applied pure tea tree oil to her scalp. It burned and made her itch worse. Once we diluted it in jojoba oil, it worked like magic.

## How to Use Oils & Butters Without Overdoing It

- Always apply on top of water or a water-based product (like leave-in).
- Start small — a pea-sized amount of butter or a few drops of oil is usually enough.
- Adjust by season: heavier oils and butters in winter, lighter ones in summer.

**Trick:** If your hair feels greasy but still dry, you're sealing without adding moisture first. Always hydrate before sealing.

## Takeaways

- Moisturizing oils (olive, avocado, coconut) penetrate for softness.
- Sealing oils (castor, jojoba, grapeseed) lock in hydration.
- Butters (shea, mango, cocoa) coat and protect — heavy but powerful.
- Essential oils are strong boosters — always dilute them.
- Oils and butters seal moisture, they don't create it.

# 13

# Protecting Your Hair in Daily Life

You can have the best wash day routine in the world, but if your daily habits are rough on your hair, the progress won't last. Think of it like fitness: you can crush the gym for an hour, but if you eat junk the rest of the day, you won't see results. Protecting your hair daily is what keeps the work you've already done from going to waste.

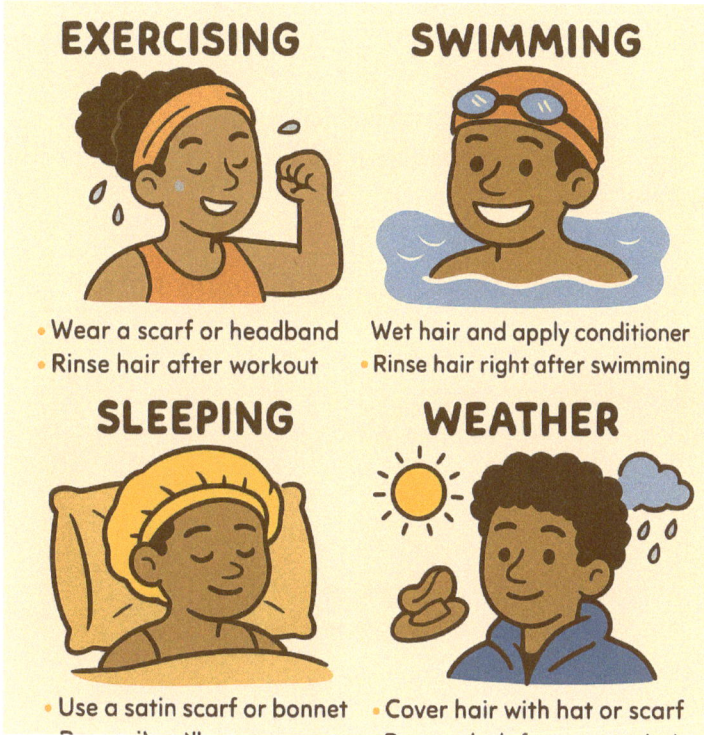

## EXERCISING
- Wear a scarf or headband
- Rinse hair after workout

## SWIMMING
Wet hair and apply conditioner
- Rinse hair right after swimming

## SLEEPING
- Use a satin scarf or bonnet

## WEATHER
- Cover hair with hat or scarf

## Exercise — Sweat Happens

Sweat itself isn't bad for your hair. It's just salty water. But left sitting on the scalp, it can cause dryness or buildup.

- **Quick fixes:**
- Rinse or refresh with water after workouts.
- Use a light leave-in spray to keep hair hydrated.
- If you wear protective styles, make sure your scalp can still breathe.

**Story:** A client once told me she skipped workouts because she "didn't want to ruin her hair." I showed her how to do quick rinses and tie her hair in a breathable scarf while exercising. She got back in the gym and kept her hair healthy.

   **Tip:** Don't let your hair stop you from moving your body. Healthy lifestyle = healthy hair, too.

## Swimming — Guarding Against Chlorine and Salt

Pools and oceans are tough. Chlorine strips the hair, and salt pulls moisture out. Think of it like leaving plants in direct sun without water — they dry out fast.

**Before swimming:**

- Wet your hair with clean water.
- Coat it with conditioner or a light oil.
- Wear a swim cap if possible.

**After swimming:**

- Rinse immediately.
- Use a gentle shampoo or clarifier.
- Follow with a deep conditioner.

**Trick:** Keep a travel-size spray bottle with conditioner and water in your bag. Use it right after swimming before you get home.

## Night Care — Protecting While You Sleep

Nighttime can undo all your hard work if you're not careful. Cotton pillowcases suck moisture out and cause friction, leading to breakage.

- **Best options:**
- Satin or silk pillowcases, bonnets, or scarves.
- Pineapple (loose ponytail) for curls to prevent flattening.
- Braids or twists to keep tangles away overnight.

**Story:** One of my clients used to wake up with her hair matted every morning. Switching to a satin pillowcase changed everything — less tangling, less dryness, and her wash days got easier.

   **Tip:** If bonnets or scarves slide off at night, double up: a satin pillowcase under your regular case is backup protection.

## Day-to-Day Habits — The Small Things Add Up

It's not just workouts and swimming. Everyday habits matter, too.

- **Weather:** Cover your hair in harsh sun, cold wind, or rain.
- **Accessories:** Use scrunchies instead of tight elastics.
- **Hands off:** Constantly touching or pulling at your hair causes frizz and breakage.
- **Rotate styles:** Don't wear the same tight bun or ponytail every day.

**Truth:** Protecting your hair doesn't mean you can't style it. It just means styling smart so your hair lasts longer and stays healthier.

## Takeaways

- Sweat isn't the enemy; buildup is. Refresh after workouts.
- Protect your hair before and after swimming with water, conditioner, and rinses.
- Night care matters — friction and dryness happen while you sleep.
- Everyday choices — weather, accessories, styling — make or break your progress.

# 14

# Locs

## A Different Kind of Garden

Locs are like vines growing into strong ropes. They take patience, consistency, and the right kind of care. Some people think locs mean "low maintenance," but really they're about **different maintenance**. When cared for properly, locs become one of the most beautiful and resilient forms of hair expression.

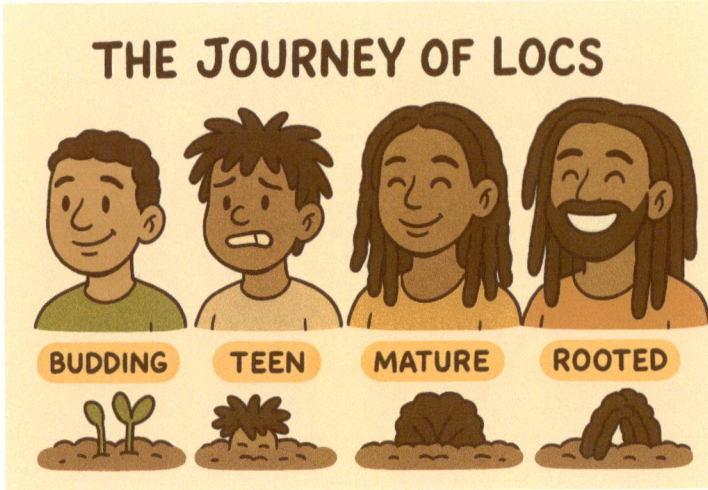

## The Growth Phases — From Budding to Mature

Locs don't form overnight. Just like plants take time to grow roots, locs go through stages.

1. **Budding Stage:** Hair begins to coil and clump together. It's fuzzy, and that's normal.
2. **Teen Stage:** Locs start to take shape but can look messy. Patience is key here.
3. **Mature Stage:** Locs are solid, with less frizz. They hold their shape and weight.
4. **Rooted Stage:** Fully developed locs with thickness, strength, and length.

**Story:** A client once panicked when her starter locs frizzed up. She thought something went wrong. I explained, "Frizz is part of the process — it means your hair is locking." Once she embraced it, she stopped fighting the fuzz and her locs flourished.

## Washing Locs — Clean Soil, Strong Roots

Some people avoid washing locs, afraid they'll unravel. But dirty scalp = unhealthy locs. Locs need clean soil to thrive.

- **How to wash:**
- Use a clarifying shampoo occasionally to remove buildup.
- Focus on the scalp, rinse thoroughly.
- Squeeze locs gently to release water — don't twist them like a towel.

**Tip:** Always dry locs fully after washing. Damp locs can trap odor and mildew. Air-dry or use a hooded dryer if needed.

## Moisture and Hydration — Keeping Locs Alive

Locs may look tough, but they can get dry inside. The trick is to moisturize without heavy buildup.

- **Best options:**
- Water-based sprays.
- Light leave-ins or rosewater.
- A touch of oil on the scalp or ends.
- **Avoid:** Heavy creams, waxes, or thick butters that get stuck inside the locs.

**Trick:** Mix water with a few drops of oil in a spray bottle for a quick daily refresher.

## Retwisting and Maintenance — Don't Overdo It

Locs need maintenance, but too much retwisting can thin out the roots and cause breakage.

- **How often:** Every 4–8 weeks, depending on hair type and growth.
- **Gentle approach:** Twist just enough to keep locs neat, not painfully tight.
- **Alternative:** Some prefer interlocking (looping the hair through itself), but moderation is still key.

**Story:** One client insisted on retwisting every two weeks. Over time, her roots weakened and her locs thinned. We switched her to monthly retwists, focused on scalp health, and her locs grew back stronger.

## Lint and Buildup — The Hidden Enemy

Locs attract lint and hold onto products if you're not careful.

- **Prevention:** Sleep with a satin scarf or bonnet, especially on light-colored sheets.
- **Avoid:** Heavy waxes, butters, and thick gels. They get trapped inside and are hard to remove.
- **Fix:** Occasional clarifying wash or an apple cider vinegar rinse can help reset.

## Everyday Care — Protecting Locs

- **Sleep:** Wrap with satin or silk to prevent lint and dryness.
- **Lint patrol:** Dark clothes, hoodies, and blankets can sneak lint into your locs. Cover hair or choose fabrics carefully.
- **Styling:** Locs are versatile, but avoid heavy updos every day — they can strain roots.

**Tip:** If you notice white fuzz inside your locs, it's usually lint, not dandruff. Prevention (satin wraps, regular washing) is easier than removal.

## Takeaways

- Locs form in stages: budding, teen, mature, rooted. Fuzz is normal.
- Wash regularly and dry thoroughly to avoid buildup and odor.
- Moisturize lightly with sprays and oils, not heavy creams.
- Retwist in moderation — overdoing it weakens roots.
- Protect locs daily with satin at night and smart styling choices.

# 15

# Risks & Potential Issues

## When Good Hair Care Goes Wrong

Even with the best products and routines, things can backfire if you overdo it or miss the balance. Healthy hair is about *consistency*, not extremes. Let's break down the common risks people run into and how to fix them.

## Product Overload — Too Much of a Good Thing

Imagine watering a plant every hour. Instead of thriving, it drowns. Hair works the same way. Piling on too many products smothers strands instead of helping.

- **Signs:** Hair feels greasy, sticky, or stiff no matter what you do. White flakes or film show up after styling.
- **Fix:** Do a clarifying wash to reset, then stick to fewer products (leave-in, cream, oil is enough).

**Story:** A client once brought me a bag of 12 different creams and gels she layered daily. Her hair felt heavy and lifeless. Once we cut her routine down to 3 core products, her curls popped again.

## Over-Oiling — Grease Isn't Growth

Oil is great for sealing, but too much clogs the scalp and attracts dirt. More oil doesn't equal faster growth.

- **Signs:** Scalp feels itchy or suffocated, hair looks shiny but still dry.
- **Fix:** Use oil only after adding moisture. Massage a few drops into the scalp — don't pour it on.

**Tip:** Think of oil as lotion for hair, not water. You still need hydration first.

## Protein Overload — Turning Hair into Straw

Protein strengthens hair, but too much makes it stiff and brittle. It's like adding too many boards to a fence — it stops bending and just breaks.

- **Signs:** Hair feels hard, crunchy, or breaks easily after protein use.
- **Fix:** Balance with moisture. Use a moisturizing deep conditioner to soften.

## Heat Overuse — The Silent Damage

Flat irons, blow dryers, and curling wands can smooth hair beautifully, but constant use fries the cuticle.

- **Signs:** Curls won't bounce back, hair looks stringy or straight when wet.
- **Fix:** Cut back on heat. Deep condition weekly. Trim off permanently damaged ends.

**Story:** A client who straightened her hair twice a week came in upset that her curls "disappeared." We had to cut the heat-damaged ends and start fresh.

## Ingredient Sensitivities — When Products Fight You

Some ingredients just don't agree with certain scalps.

- **Sulfates:** Great cleansers, but drying if overused.
- **Fragrance:** Can cause itchiness or irritation.
- **Heavy Butters/Waxes:** Can clog fine strands or locs.

**Tip:** If your scalp suddenly starts itching or burning, don't ignore it — check the label. Switch to fragrance-free or gentler formulas.

## Neglect — The Biggest Risk of All

Skipping trims, ignoring wash day, or never moisturizing might not show damage right away, but it adds up. It's like skipping dentist visits — problems grow quietly until they're big.

94

- **Signs:** Chronic dryness, endless tangles, breakage.
- **Fix:** Stick to the basics: wash, condition, moisturize, protect. Simplicity beats neglect every time.

## Takeaways

- Too many products weigh hair down — less is more.
- Oil seals moisture; it doesn't replace it.
- Balance protein and moisture to keep hair flexible.
- Heat overuse causes permanent damage — protect and limit it.
- Pay attention to ingredient sensitivities — your scalp always tells the truth.
- Consistency matters more than chasing miracle fixes.

# 16

# Red Flags vs. Green Lights

Let's keep it real: your hair talks to you. Sometimes it's whispering,

**"We're good, keep doing that."** Other times it's yelling, **"Stop, you're hurting me!"**

The problem is, most people don't know how to tell the difference. So let's break it down — what's a **red flag** and what's a **green light** when it comes to your routine.

## Red Flags — When Your Hair Is Crying For Help

- **Your scalp is always itchy after you use a product.** That's not "just how your scalp is." It's your skin telling you it doesn't like what's in that bottle — usually fragrance or a harsh ingredient.
- **Your hair feels coated, waxy, or greasy no matter what you do.** That's product buildup. Oils, silicones, and butters are sitting on top instead of sinking in. Time for a reset with a

clarifying shampoo.

· **Your ends keep splitting even though you trim.** That's because you're moisturizing but not sealing. Think of it like watering a plant but never putting soil on top — the water just evaporates.

· **Your hair snaps when you detangle.** If every comb-through sounds like a battle, your products aren't giving you enough slip. Detangling should feel smooth, not stressful.

· **Your styles flop within hours.** If your twist-out or wash-and-go falls apart before the day is done, it could be buildup, the wrong product for your climate, or just too much layering.

· **You're using six different bottles just to style once.** That's not a routine — that's product overload. More isn't better, it's just more.

## Green Lights — When You Know You're Winning

· **Detangling feels easy.** Your comb glides, your fingers slip through, and you're not losing a handful of hair.

· **Your hair feels soft and bouncy, not heavy.** That means you've hit that sweet spot between moisture and protein.

· **Your scalp feels calm and clean.** No itching, no tightness, no flakes. It's breathing.

· **Day 2 hair actually looks better than Day 1.** That's a sign your products are working with your hair, not against it.

· **You're using fewer products and getting better results.** When your shelf is simple but your hair is thriving, that's the win.

· **Your hair is not just growing, but staying.** You're retaining length, trims are light, and your ends look healthy.

# RED FLAGS

⚠ Scalp always itchy after a product

⚠ Hair feels coated or waxy no matter what

⚠ Ends keep splitting even with trims

⚠ Hair breaks during detangling

⚠ Styles flop within hours

⚠ Spending more time layering products than actually styling

# GREEN LIGHTS

✓ Detangling feels easy

✓ Hair feels soft and bouncy – not heavy

✓ Scalp feels calm and clean

✓ Day 2 hair looks better than Day 1

✓ You're using fewer products, but getting better results

✓ Hair grows out and actually stays

## Story From the Chair

I once had a client come in and say, "I need six products to make my curls behave." I asked her, "If your hair needs six referees, maybe the problem isn't the curls." We stripped her routine down to a leave-in, an oil, and one gel. She came back the next week grinning, "This is the softest my hair has *ever* been." Sometimes less really is more.

## The Bottom Line

Red Flags mean your hair is trying to warn you. Green Lights mean you're finally in the groove. The key is paying attention, making small tweaks, and trusting what your hair is showing you. Because at the end of the day, the best routine isn't the one with the fanciest bottles — it's the one that actually works for *you*.

# 17

# Growth and Retention

## Keeping What You Grow

Here's the truth: your hair is always growing. The real challenge isn't growth — it's retention. You can sprout inches from the scalp, but if your ends keep breaking off, you'll never see the length. Think of it like filling a bucket with a hole at the bottom. You can pour all the water you want in, but unless you patch the hole, it'll never stay full.

## Growth — The Scalp's Job

Your scalp and follicles handle growth on their own, as long as they're healthy.

- **Blood flow = nutrients.** Massage your scalp, stay hydrated, and eat well.
- **Healthy scalp = strong roots.** Keep it clean and balanced, not clogged with oils or products.

- **Cycles matter.** Anagen (growth) lasts years, Catagen (transition) lasts weeks, Telogen (rest/shedding) lasts months. Shedding is natural — don't panic.

**Tip:** Growth starts from the inside. Stress, poor diet, and lack of sleep can slow it down.

## Retention — Your Job

Retention is about protecting the hair that's already out of your head. This is where most people lose the battle.

- **Moisturize and Seal:** Hydrate regularly and lock it in. Dry hair breaks fast.
- **Protective Styling:** Braids, twists, buns, wigs, and locs protect ends from friction and breakage.
- **Trim on Time:** Split ends don't repair — they spread. Trim every 8–12 weeks.
- **Gentle Handling:** Finger detangle or use wide-tooth combs. Rough detangling = snapped strands.

**Story:** A client once told me, "My hair hasn't grown in years." I showed her her new growth near the roots — it was there. The problem was her ends were breaking just as fast. Once she started moisturizing consistently and protecting her ends, she saw inches of growth for the first time in years.

## Lifestyle Habits That Support Growth

- **Nutrition:** Protein, iron, omega-3s, and vitamins all play a role.
- **Hydration:** Water feeds your follicles from the inside.
- **Exercise:** Boosts blood circulation to the scalp.
- **Sleep:** Your body repairs and grows while you rest.

**Tip:** Treat hair health like body health. A strong body grows strong hair.

## Myths That Block Progress

- **"Oil makes hair grow faster."** Oil seals — it doesn't sprout new strands.
- **"Trimming makes hair grow."** Trimming doesn't speed growth, it prevents breakage so you see the growth you already have.
- **"Protective styles guarantee growth."** They help retain length, but if you don't moisturize underneath, damage still happens.

## Quick Tricks for Retention

- Sleep on satin or silk.
- Keep ends tucked in styles when possible.
- Moisturize lightly every other day or as needed.
- Avoid constant manipulation — the less you fuss, the more you retain.

## Takeaways

- Growth happens naturally at the scalp if you're healthy inside and out.
- Retention is the real battle — protect ends, moisturize, seal, and trim.
- Healthy lifestyle habits (food, water, sleep, exercise) directly affect hair growth.
- Myths can distract you — focus on consistency and protection.
- Retention is what turns growth into visible length.

# 18

# Myths vs Facts

The Truth About Hair

# MYTHS vs. FACTS
## THE TRUTH ABOUT HAIR

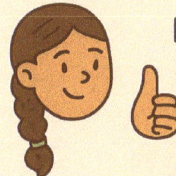

| MYTH | FACT |
|---|---|
| Trimming makes your hair grow faster. | Trims help **PROTECT** length. |
| Oil makes hair grow. | Care for hair underneath. |
| Protective styles moiturizer. | True moisture comes from water. |
| More product = better results | Less is more. |
| | Natural hair is manageable |

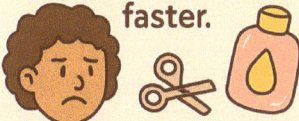

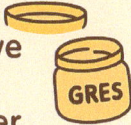

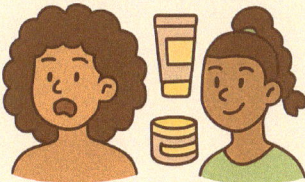

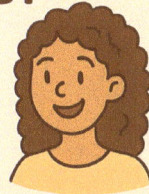

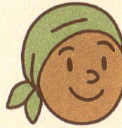

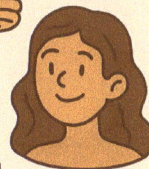

## Myth 1: "Trimming makes your hair grow faster."

**Story:** A client once said she skipped trims because she wanted long hair. But every time her hair grew, the split ends crept up and broke off.

   **Fact:** Trims don't make hair *grow* faster — they help you *keep* the length you already have.

## Myth 2: "Oil makes hair grow."

**Analogy:** Pouring oil on the outside of a plant won't make it sprout faster — the growth happens in the roots. Same with your scalp.

   **Fact:** Oil seals in moisture and nourishes the scalp, but hair growth comes from blood flow, nutrition, and healthy follicles.

## Myth 3: "Protective styles guarantee growth."

**Story:** Someone wore braids back-to-back for a year and expected inches of growth. Instead, she faced breakage when she never moisturized underneath.

   **Fact:** Protective styles help retain length, but only if you still care for your scalp and hair underneath.

## Myth 4: "Grease is the best moisturizer."

**Analogy:** Grease is like plastic wrap. If your hair is already dry, it just locks dryness in.

   **Fact:** True moisture comes from water and water-based products. Oils and butters *seal* that moisture in — they don't replace it.

## Myth 5: "More product = better results."

**Story:** A client layered five creams, two gels, and oil daily. Her curls felt heavy, sticky, and dull.

**Fact:** Less is more. The right product in the right amount always beats overload.

## Myth 6: "Natural hair is unmanageable."

**Analogy:** Untamed grass looks wild, but with watering and trimming, it's beautiful. Same with natural hair — it just needs routine.

**Fact:** Natural hair is versatile and manageable when you use the right methods and patience.

### Takeaways

- Trims protect, they don't speed growth.
- Oils seal, they don't sprout hair.
- Protective styles help only if you care underneath.
- Moisture = water, not grease.
- Less product = more results.
- Natural hair is manageable with consistency.

# 19

# Tips & Tricks

## The Little Things That Make a Big Difference

Sometimes it's not about doing more for your hair — it's about doing the right small things consistently. These tips and tricks save time, prevent damage, and make hair care feel less like a chore and more like a lifestyle.

# TiPS & TrickS

**TRIM TO PROTECT LENGTH**

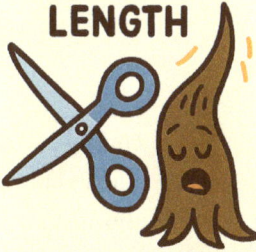

**REFRESH WITH WATER + LEAVE-IN = INSTANT LIFE**

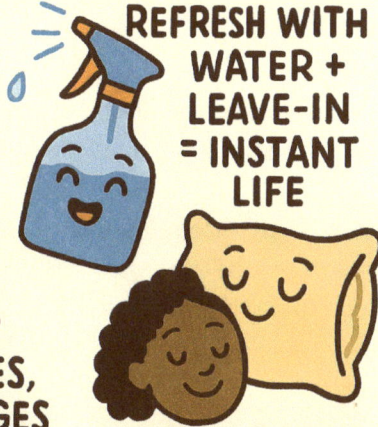

**ROTATE STYLES, SAVE YOUR EDGES**

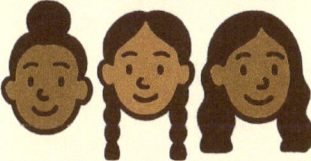

**TRAVEL KIT**
YOUR HAIR'S CARRY-ON ESSENTIALS

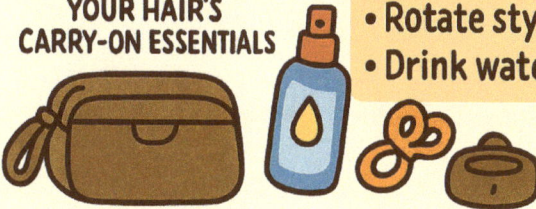

**Cheat SHEET**
- Sleep on satin
- Moisturize lightly
- Trim ends
- Rotate styles
- Drink water

## Trim Smart, Not Scared

Split ends spread like cracks in a windshield. A tiny snip now saves inches later.

- **Tip:** Trim every 8–12 weeks or whenever ends feel rough and snag.
- **Trick:** Search-and-destroy method — trim single-strand knots instead of waiting for a full cut.

**Story:** A client once refused trims for a year, hoping to keep her length. By the time she came back, the splits had climbed halfway up her strands. We had to cut much more than she wanted. She learned trims actually protect length.

## Master the Spray Bottle

A spray bottle is your best friend. Fill it with water and a bit of leave-in conditioner for a quick refresh.

- **Tip:** Mist lightly — don't drench.
- **Trick:** Add a drop of oil to the mix for extra shine and softness.

## Satin = Secret Weapon

Friction kills moisture. Cotton pillowcases act like sponges, pulling hydration out of your hair.

- **Tip:** Sleep with satin or silk pillowcases, bonnets, or scarves.
- **Trick:** If bonnets slip off, double up — bonnet + satin

pillowcase.

## Style Rotation — Save Your Edges

Wearing the same tight bun, ponytail, or braids every day stresses your edges.

- **Tip:** Rotate styles weekly.
- **Trick:** Use tension-free styles when you know you'll be busy or working out.

## Quick Refresh Recipe

Mix water, leave-in conditioner, and a few drops of oil in a spray bottle. Shake and spray for instant moisture.

- **Tip:** Keep a travel-size bottle in your bag.
- **Trick:** Add aloe juice for extra hydration.

## Workout and Swim Hacks

- **Before workouts:** Wrap hair loosely in a scarf to minimize frizz.
- **After workouts:** Rinse scalp or mist with refresher spray.
- **Before swimming:** Wet hair with clean water and coat with conditioner.
- **After swimming:** Rinse immediately and deep condition later.

## Know Your Porosity Cheat Sheet

- **Low Porosity:** Use steam or heat to open cuticles. Stick to lighter products.
- **Medium Porosity:** Most products work — just don't overload.
- **High Porosity:** Layer products and always seal with oils or butters.

## Travel Kit Must-Haves

- Mini satin pillowcase
- Travel-size leave-in
- Wide-tooth comb
- Scrunchies or spiral ties
- Small oil bottle

**Trick:** This kit keeps your routine alive even on vacation or at a friend's place.

## Takeaways

- Small, consistent habits save length and prevent damage.
- A spray bottle mix is the cheapest, easiest refresher.
- Satin at night = moisture protection.
- Rotate styles to protect your edges.
- Simple hacks for workouts, swimming, and travel keep your hair thriving anywhere.

# 20

# Pulling It All Together

## Your Healthy Hair Routine

By now, you've learned the science, the stories, and the steps. But knowledge means nothing without action. This chapter gives you simple routines and checklists to put everything into motion. Think of it as your personal playbook — something you can return to again and again.

## The Weekly Wash-Day Routine

1. **Detangle** — Mist hair with water or leave-in, gently work through knots from ends to roots.
2. **Wash** — Use moisturizing shampoo most weeks, clarifying once a month. Focus on scalp, not ends.
3. **Condition** — Always condition. Deep condition weekly for extra nourishment.
4. **Seal** — Apply oil or butter after moisturizing to lock in hydration.

5. **Protect** — Style in a way that keeps ends tucked or edges safe.
6. **Moisturize (between washes)** — Refresh with a light mist of water + leave-in.

**Trick:** Break your wash day into steps with breaks in between. Detangle in the morning, wash midday, style at night. No rush = less stress.

## The Daily Quick-Care Routine

- **Morning**: Light mist of water/leave-in if needed, style loosely.
- **During the day:** Hands off — the less you touch, the less frizz.
- **Night:** Satin pillowcase, bonnet, or scarf. Twist or pineapple to protect curls.

**Tip:** Listen to your hair. If it feels rough, add moisture. If it feels soft but limp, balance with protein.

## Monthly Reset Routine

- Clarify with a deep cleanser.
- Follow with a protein treatment to strengthen.
- Deep condition with moisture to balance.
- Trim ends if needed.

## Growth & Retention Checklist

- Massage scalp 1–2 times a week.
- Drink water daily.
- Eat balanced meals (protein, iron, vitamins).
- Limit tight styles — edges matter.
- Stick to trims every 8–12 weeks.

**Truth:** Growth happens naturally, but retention is earned through care.

## Loc Routine (For Readers with Locs)

- Wash every 1–3 weeks, dry fully.
- Mist with rosewater or aloe spray daily.
- Retwist every 4–8 weeks, not tighter.
- Sleep in satin to avoid lint.
- Avoid heavy waxes or creams.

## Final Words of Encouragement

Healthy hair isn't about chasing products or copying trends. It's about **consistency, balance, and patience**. Just like a garden, your hair thrives when you feed the soil, water regularly, and protect it from harm.
   **Remember:**

- The Secret 6 Steps are your foundation.
- Balance moisture and protein.
- Protect daily, trim when needed.
- Love your unique texture — it tells your story.

**Pro Tip:** Don't compare your hair journey to anyone else's. Focus on progress, not perfection. Every inch you keep is a win.

## Takeaways

- Weekly, daily, and monthly routines keep hair balanced and thriving.
- Growth is natural, retention is the goal.
- Locs require unique but simple care: light moisture, clean scalp, protection.
- Consistency beats every "miracle product."
- Healthy hair is a lifestyle, not a one-time fix.

KOY.KUT
MASTER BARBER

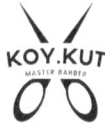

# About the Author

**Koy Kut** is a master barber, entrepreneur, and educator with a passion for helping people feel confident from the inside out. Known for his precision cuts and creative approach to natural hair, Koy has spent years studying not just styles, but the *science* behind healthy hair.

Through his work behind the chair, Koy saw a pattern — people were taking care of their hair without actually understanding it. That inspired him to create educational content and resources that simplify the process, making healthy hair care something anyone can master.

His philosophy is simple: **"Knowledge first, products second."** When you understand your scalp, your texture, and your routine, you stop chasing trends and start building results that last.

Koy is also the author of *Hair on the Mind: The Connection Between Hair and Mental Health* and *Confident Cut: How Hair Can Teach You Confidence.* Across all his work, his message stays the same — that hair isn't just about appearance, it's about identity, discipline, and self-expression.

When he's not in the shop, Koy continues to educate through writing, workshops, and digital projects designed to empower the next generation of barbers, stylists, and everyday people to take control of their hair journeys.

# Also by Koy Kut

*Hair on the Mind: The Connection Between Hair and Mental Health*

An honest exploration of how self-image, confidence, and culture are deeply tied to the way we see our hair — and how caring for it can become an act of healing.

*Confident Cut: How Hair Can Teach You Confidence*

A motivational guide that uses the barber chair as a classroom, showing how self-discipline, appearance, and mindset work together to build real confidence.

*The Hair Type Handbook: Everything You Need to Know to Love Your Hair*

A fun, educational guide to understanding your texture, porosity, and curl pattern — designed to help readers embrace their natural hair without confusion or comparison.

*Our Hair, Our Story*

A cultural journey through the history, meaning, and power of hair in the Black community — celebrating identity, resilience, and style through every strand.

www.ingramcontent.com/pod-product-compliance
Lightning Source LLC
Chambersburg PA
CBHW040128270326
41927CB00004B/90